Drugs
of **Abuse**

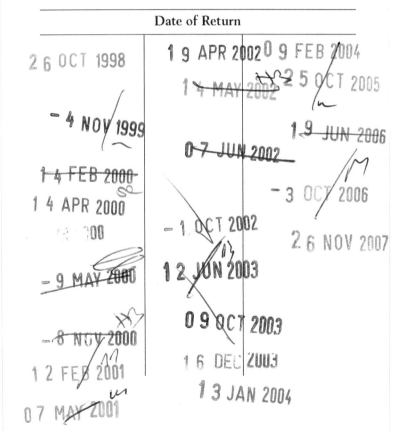
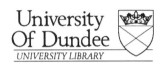

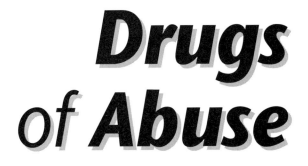

Drugs
of Abuse

Simon Wills

MSc, MRPharmS

Head of Drug Information
Portsmouth Hospitals NHS Trust

The Pharmaceutical Press

Published by The Pharmaceutical Press
1 Lambeth High Street, London SE1 7JN

First published 1997

Typeset by Florencetype Ltd, Stoodleigh, Devon
Printed in Great Britain at the University Press, Cambridge

ISBN 0 85369 352 8

A catalogue record for this book is available from the
British Library.

All photographs by the author except Figure 17.1
(Royal Pharmaceutical Society Library) and Figure 16.3
(Peter Houghton, King's College, London).

To Mum, Dad, Richard,
Jonathan and Mike

Simon Wills

Simon Wills studied for a degree in pharmacy at King's College, London University, before qualifying as a pharmacist in 1988. He has been Head of Drug Information at Portsmouth Hospitals NHS Trust since completing an MSc in Clinical Pharmacy in 1991. He is currently studying the pharmacoepidemiology of adverse drug reactions for a PhD at Portsmouth University. His interest in drugs of abuse was stimulated by awareness of an increasing need for clinical information about drug abuse and its consequences by healthcare professionals. Establishment of a database in Portsmouth has led to an increasing demand for information from around the country. He has now written widely on the subject.

Contents

Preface

Whether we approve of drug abuse wholly, selectively or not at all, it has been with the human race since before the dawn of written history and is here to stay. This book aims to be a detailed handbook for the healthcare professional who works with drug users or who wants to know more about the subject in an easily digestible form. I have tried to be concise but clear, so that the book is small, relevant, easy to read and relatively cheap. I want the book above all to be useful: as an educational tool, a clinical resource or a reference. I welcome comments from readers on the content or presentation of the book.

The biggest problem that I had in writing this book was finding the time to write. In this respect I owe an enormous debt to all those close to me for understanding how limited my time had become and how important the book was to me. I want to say how grateful I am to them all for putting up with me being so antisocial; they are: Mum and Dad, my brother Richard, Jonathan, Mike, Jonathan and Catharine, Aileen, Tabitha, Mike A., Sarah and Henry, Manjo, Kate and Nick, Andy and Jane and many others.

I would particularly like to thank Barbara Pitman and Pauline Morris from the library at St Mary's Hospital Portsmouth for their assistance in obtaining references. Nothing has been too much trouble and I am very grateful for their help. I also want to thank Jo Lumb at the Royal Pharmaceutical Society, who gave me so much support when I first started writing about drug abuse for *The Pharmaceutical Journal*; Dave Brown at the University of Portsmouth who, apart from being the most patient PhD tutor in the world, first came up with the idea of writing this book; Paul Weller and John Wilson at the Pharmaceutical Press for making the book possible, and for not sticking too closely to deadlines; Norman Feerick (Havant) and Anne Hodge (Southampton) from the Drugs Squad who kindly enabled me to photograph many drugs of abuse and, finally, my colleagues in the pharmacy department, Portsmouth Hospitals NHS Trust who, like others, are probably heartily sick of hearing me go on about this book.

1

Introduction

'Where shall I begin, please your Majesty?' he asked.
'Begin at the beginning' the King said, gravely, 'and
go on till you come to the end: then stop.'
Lewis Carroll, 'Alice's Adventures in Wonderland'.

This chapter defines some of the terms which will be used frequently throughout the book, explains the methods of drug administration and describes the UK law related to drug abuse.

DEFINITIONS

Abuse

Abuse and dependence are distinctly different concepts, although as far as street drugs are concerned, the former must occur before the latter. The term 'abuse' is often used to describe non-medical self-administration of a substance to produce psychoactive effects, intoxication or altered body image, and usually despite knowledge of potential adverse effects. This is how the term is used in this book. Abuse can be experimental (the initial exploration of effects) or recreational (occasional or regular use without dependence).

In the USA, the Diagnostic and Statistical Manual of Mental Disorders (DSM) endorses the fact that abuse and dependence are different [1]. According to the criteria laid down in the DSM for diagnosis of abuse the individual must satisfy at least one of the following signs recurrently because of drug usage:

- failure to fulfil important personal commitments;
- abuse of drug in physically hazardous situations;

- legal problems related to abuse;
- problems in relating to other people due to abuse.

This is a rather rigid classification which concentrates on the social consequences for the individual rather than the purpose of abuse. The DSM definition of abuse is an American one; in the UK this kind of behaviour would usually be termed 'problem drug taking'.

The term 'drug abuse' is viewed by some as inappropriate because it can be seen as judgemental. However, alternatives are not very satisfactory. 'Drug use' is bland and fails to separate medicinal agent from recreational drug. 'Drug misuse' tends to imply that a drug has a proper use and is being employed for an incorrect purpose. For many illicit substances there are no 'correct' uses – the sole use is as a psychoactive drug. 'Misuse' may be a more appropriate term for the taking of over-the-counter and prescription medicines for psychoactive effects, as this constitutes incorrect use of a preparation intended as a medicinal product. Most dictionaries, however, make little distinction between the definition of abuse and misuse.

Dependence

Dependence is an inappropriate compulsion to take a substance regularly which may cause physical, mental and/or behavioural impairment. It is equivalent to the older term 'addiction', but dependence is now preferred because it is less emotive. According to the DSM criteria [1], at least three of the following must be satisfied over a 12-month period to qualify as true dependence:

1. The user shows tolerance.
2. The user suffers withdrawal – the withdrawal syndrome appears or there is clear evidence of negative reinforcement.
3. The quantity taken and/or the duration of the habit exceed the initial expectations of the user.
4. The user consistently wishes to reduce or control substance use and may have already tried to, unsuccessfully.
5. Drug-seeking behaviour and/or postexposure recovery take up a significant amount of the user's time.
6. Important personal activities are given little time or are abandoned.
7. Use of the substance continues despite the user experiencing harm from it.

Physiological (physical) dependence would be diagnosed if the user met three of these criteria, including one or both of the first two criteria.

The last five criteria (3–7) largely constitute elements of what used to be called psychological dependence.

Designer drugs

Dr Gary Henderson from the University of California introduced this term to describe analogues of street drugs that were manufactured in order to circumvent the law [2]. Ecstasy and other amphetamine analogues were being synthesised and used legally in the USA because their structures were not specified as illicit substances in the legislation of the time.

The term has now acquired a different meaning because current legal specifications for illicit substances in the USA and UK are so detailed that circumventing the law is very difficult. A designer drug, in the most popular use of the term, is an analogue of an existing well-known street drug, with similar pharmacological properties but a different chemical structure [3]. It is therefore a very imprecise term. Substances referred to as designer drugs include analogues of fentanyl, methamphetamine, pethidine and phencyclidine.

The term 'designer drug' should not be taken to imply that an analogue can be synthesised or prepared to meet an individual's requirement (i.e. akin to 'designer clothes'). This is not possible.

Drug-seeking behaviour

Those with a compulsion to take an abusable substance may go to great lengths to obtain further supplies. This may include regularly buying the drug, theft (of the drug, or money to buy it), forgery of prescriptions, selling valuable possessions in order to obtain drugs and prioritising drug-seeking above other more urgent matters.

Intoxication

This is a characteristic pattern of behavioural, mental and physical changes caused by the administration of a psychoactive drug. The DSM criteria [1] describe the changes induced by intoxication as 'maladaptive', i.e. inappropriate to the social or environmental setting and may place the individual at risk of harm. Broadly, the nature of intoxication is similar in individuals that ingest the same drug; the detailed effects differ depending on a variety of factors. Some of the most important factors are: dose, method of administration, state of mind, the environment and drug handling by the body. Intoxication abates gradually as a drug is eliminated.

Reinforcement

Both positive and negative reinforcement exist. When the pleasurable effects of drug-taking are the main cause of repeated administration, this is termed positive reinforcement. Each time a dose is taken the desired effects are produced, reinforcing the desire to take more drug.

When the main drive behind repeated administration is the desire to avoid or reverse a withdrawal reaction, this is called negative reinforcement. Whenever the drug is taken, the individual manages to stave off the unpleasantness of withdrawal for a bit longer.

Tolerance

This occurs when repeated administration of a drug eventually produces a reduced effect, such that larger doses are required to achieve the same response.

Withdrawal reaction

This is a collection of signs and symptoms which occur if the dose of a drug is reduced suddenly, if an antagonist is given or if administration is stopped abruptly. Sustained heavy administration of a drug on a regular basis for a number of weeks is usually required before such a state can be precipitated. The reaction has a finite duration, although duration and exact symptomatology may vary widely between individuals. Some individuals do not appear to experience withdrawal reactions, despite pursuing a pattern of administration which would lead one to assume that such a reaction should occur. There may be an acute phase which is relatively brief (days) and occurs shortly after dosage reduction or cessation, and a chronic phase which succeeds this and lasts much longer (months). Both acute and chronic phases may be associated with craving for the drug.

THE LAW AND DRUG ABUSE

Legal status of drugs

In the UK, drugs of abuse are controlled by two main pieces of legislation.

Misuse of Drugs Act (1971)

This Act classifies drugs into three classes according to the maximum penalty which an offender can expect to receive if he or she contravenes the law. The Act renders possession, export, import, manufacture or supply of any of these drugs illegal except in certain specified circumstances.

Class A drugs   Pure cannabinoids (but not cannabis itself), cocaine, LSD, opioids, phencyclidine, psilocybin. Injectable forms of drugs in class B.

Class B drugs   Amphetamine, barbiturates, cannabis, codeine, dihydrocodeine, ecstasy, methamphetamine, methylphenidate.

Class C drugs   Benzodiazepines, cathine, cathinone, dextropropoxyphene, diethylpropion, anabolic steroids, human chorionic gonadotrophin and growth hormones.

Misuse of Drugs Regulations (1985)

These are principally concerned with regulating the legitimate supply and use of abusable substances.

Schedule 1 (CD Lic)   Only those persons licensed by the Home Office may possess or supply these drugs. None of them can be prescribed. The drugs in this schedule are those deemed to have little therapeutic value and so licences are usually only issued for research purposes. The drugs involved include cannabis, cannabinol, cathinone, ecstasy and related drugs, designer opioids derived from fentanyl (but not fentanyl itself), LSD, raw opium and coca leaf.

Schedule 2 (CD)   The Regulations give a long list of exemptions but, in most circumstances, possession of these drugs by a member of the public is only lawful when acting under the directions of a doctor. For those that supply them, the drugs are subject to stringent requirements for storage and documentation. Examples of drugs affected include amphetamine, cocaine, opioids (with certain exceptions including oral codeine and dihydrocodeine) and phencyclidine.

Schedule 3 (CD No Reg)   These are subject to the same regulations as schedule 2 except that the documentation of supply is less rigorous. Barbiturates, buprenorphine and cathine are included here.

Schedule 4 (CD Benz)   Part I contains anabolic steroids, growth hormones, human chorionic gonadotrophin and clenbuterol. Part II comprises mostly benzodiazepines.

Schedule 5 (CD Inv)   These are preparations containing very small amounts of substances which would otherwise belong to schedule 2 or 3. Examples include codeine linctus, and kaolin and morphine mixture. Suppliers and producers must keep transaction records of their dealings.

Drugs not covered

Certain abused substances are not covered by either of these two pieces of legislation. Examples include nitrites, volatile substances, over-the-counter medicines, 'smart' drugs and gamma-hydroxybutyrate.

Legalisation

The arguments surrounding the legalisation of any one, or all, of the currently illicit substances are very interesting; not least the debate on what form legalisation might take. Wholesale legalisation of production, supply and possession of all drugs is the most liberal option but there are various halfway measures. These include: allowing the sale of substances via registered premises only; decriminalising personal possession if the individual has no intent to supply; legalising possession and supply of substances manufactured under government licence only and not those from illicit sources; permitting wider supply via drug dependency clinics to registered abusers; and limiting legalisation to certain drugs only.

Without targeting a specific drug, what are the reasons for and against legalising a currently illegal substance? Some of the arguments commonly used on both sides are summarised below.

Arguments in favour of legalisation

Freedom of choice   Any individual should have the right to take any pharmacologically active agent that he or she chooses. Alcohol, tobacco and caffeine are legal substances that are known to have potentially harmful effects – why should other psychoactive substances not be freely available in a similar way? Many abusable substances are thought to be considerably less harmful than tobacco or alcohol. Some of them are legal in other countries (e.g. cannabis in The Netherlands, khat in Yemen), and others have been legal in the UK in the past (e.g. opium in England until 1868).

Quality control   Legalisation opens the door to quality control of abusable substances. This would prevent the involvement of potentially harmful contaminants, avoid accidental overdoses due to lack of knowledge of concentration and enable an individual to know exactly what he or she was taking. Injectable drugs could be supplied, correctly formulated, in sterilised ampoules, reducing the risk of injection site infection and other adverse consequences of injection (see Chapter 2). Needles and syringes would be supplied to cut down the spread of AIDS and other infections from the sharing of injection equipment.

Reduced crime   Thefts and assaults to obtain money to buy drugs would be drastically reduced if drugs were legalised and available free on the National Health Service or cheaply from agreed outlets.

Reduced profits for criminal organisations   A number of large criminal organisations generate vast sums of money by manufacturing and supplying illegal substances. All street drugs are very cheap to mass produce and are not intrinsically costly; their illegal status currently keeps street prices high. Legalisation would remove a vital source of income for criminal organisations and, with reduced revenue, this might in turn reduce their activity and influence in other areas.

Decreased workload for law enforcers   Drug abuse currently forms a large part of the workload of the police, customs, lawyers and courts. Legalising a drug reduces public expenditure in these areas and frees public servants for other duties.

Laws have not worked   Drug abuse is widespread, so the current legal controls have not worked. People who really want to abuse drugs will do so whether they are illegal or not. It is time to be more liberal in our approach and stop wasting effort on enforcing a system that has not worked.

Arguments against legalisation

The unknown   Legalisation is largely a voyage into the unknown. Arguments in favour of legalisation are rather theoretical and based on conjecture. We cannot foresee what might happen to individuals and to our society if a drug is legalised. It is not appropriate to guess what may happen in the UK based on what has happened in our own past or in other countries because each culture and era is different. It would be difficult to reverse a decision to legalise a drug if we found the effects of legalisation were not to our liking. Tobacco and alcohol do have harmful effects but they are legal substances for historical reasons; rendering both of these illegal would be extraordinarily difficult because large sections of the population that would not have taken them were they illegal would now resist criminalisation.

Adverse effects   The abusable substances that are currently illicit have never been subjected to formal clinical trials so there is insufficient information on human safety. There is little information on long-term safety for most drugs of abuse, especially with regard to central nervous system toxicity and psychiatric effects. Many drugs produce dependence, which can have great personal costs. However, it is not just the direct toxicity to the individual which can be a problem, it is the indirect effects arising from intoxication such as accidents, violence and crime. The legalisation of drugs of abuse would lead to increased usage and consequently increased health problems. Alcohol and tobacco are bad enough in terms of potential to cause ill health, unhappiness and death. Health campaigns do warn of the dangers of tobacco and alcohol but how can the government then legalise other abusable substances and so add to the problem!

Control   The current legal framework for controlling drug abuse is not perfect, but it does at least allow some control to be exerted over individuals. If new drugs of abuse were freely available, this could result in vastly increased usage and anarchy, and it might be uncontrollable.

Society's protective role   Society has a duty to protect the vulnerable who might be swept up in the use of new abusable substances. People who are young, suffering from psychiatric illness, mentally retarded, ill-educated or poor could all suffer disproportionately as a result of legalisation.

Cost   The expense of regulation, quality control and potentially increased health costs could be very great.

Philosophy of life   Individuals should not need to resort to pharmacological methods in order to enjoy life. We should try to find happiness in real life experiences.

METHODS OF ADMINISTRATION

There are three basic methods by which drugs of abuse are taken into the body: by injection, by mouth and via the airways.

Injection

Many drugs are commonly given by intravenous injection including cocaine hydrochloride, heroin, amphetamine and temazepam. The intravenous route affords rapid access to the circulation and thence to the brain, allowing fast onset of intense psychoactive effects. However, bypassing the body's normal defence mechanisms in the gut carries great risks to health. This topic is addressed more fully in Chapter 2. The subcutaneous route is an alternative which is occasionally used if the intravenous route is not available. Intra-arterial injections are usually only given by mistake when a needle misses a vein. The intramuscular route is only used for anabolic steroids.

Oral administration

For many drugs the oral route is preferred for convenience – ecstasy, LSD, alcohol and caffeine are all usually taken in this way. In addition many of the plants, smart drugs and abused medicines discussed in this book are administered by mouth. Nearly all drugs can be taken orally; this tends not to be the route of choice because many of them are absorbed from the gut unpredictably, effects can take a long time to develop and/or are blunted. Testosterone, methylphenidate, nitrites and fentanyl are examples of drugs with very poor oral bioavailability.

Administration via airways

There are several methods of exploiting the large surface area for absorption afforded by the human airways. Certain solvents, propellants and fuels can be inhaled directly into the lungs by those engaged in volatile substance abuse. Nitrites are also volatile and can be inhaled directly. Other compounds need to be heated before inhalation is possible. This is called vaporisation. Examples include heroin ('chasing the dragon'), crack cocaine, cannabis resin ('hot knifing') and methamphetamine. Smoking has a similar net effect but the drug – or drug plus an inflammable vehicle – is set alight first. Tobacco, heroin, phencyclidine and cannabis can be smoked. Some examples of home-made smoking apparatus are shown in Figure 1.1.

Dry powdered drug can be inhaled into the nose, a procedure known as 'snorting'. Amphetamine and cocaine hydrochloride are classically taken by this route.

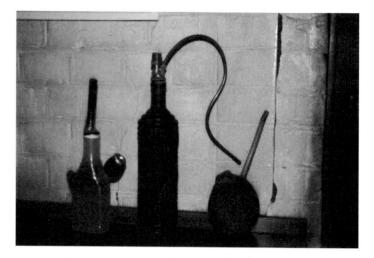

Figure 1.1 Apparatus used for smoking street drugs.
A 'lung' on the left and two 'bongs'.

REFERENCES

1.   American Psychiatric Association (1994) *DSM-IV, Diagnostic and Statistical Manual of Mental Disorders*, American Psychiatric Association, Washington, DC, pp. 175–184.
2.   Buchanan, J.F. and Brown, C.F. (1988) 'Designer drugs' – a problem in clinical toxicology. *Med. Toxicol.* **3**: 1–17.
3.   Anon. (1993) Designer drugs. *NIDA Capsule (CAP10)*, National Institute on Drug Abuse, USA, pp. 1–4.

Adverse consequences of drug injection

*Hypodermic injections should be prepared extempora-
neously. In most cases they are plain solutions of
alkaloidal or other salts in water. All utensils used
should be sterilised by thorough washing and drying
in an oven at 220 degrees Fahrenheit. The distilled
water must also be sterilised by boiling.*

Instructions for preparation of injections, in
'Pharmaceutical Formulas', 1911.

Most intravenous drug users do not start by injecting. Cocaine, amphetamine and heroin are the main drugs which are administered
intravenously, and the majority of current users who inject these drugs
began by taking them in a non-parenteral form, or started by taking
non-parenteral drugs alone. Many chronic drug abusers eventually prefer
to inject rather than administer by other routes and there are a number
of reasons for this. Intravenous administration provides the quickest
access to the circulation, resulting in rapid passage of the drug to the
brain. This produces the fastest possible onset of intoxication, and
usually a 'rush' or 'buzz' of initial euphoria occurs when a bolus of drug
reaches the brain. This effect is particularly sought after. Other methods
of administration generally provide a slower onset and a less intense
'rush'. Non-parenteral methods often involve a degree of wastage as
well: when given orally a proportion of the dose may not be absorbed
or may be metabolised by the liver before reaching the brain; smoking
or vaporisation usually destroys some of the drug; inhalation wastes the
percentage of the drug which passes down the throat to be absorbed
more slowly later.

Apart from these considerations, injecting forms part of the ritual of drug abuse for many individuals. Ritual is an important component of the injection drug user's experience – in a similar way, tobacco smokers or coffee drinkers prefer to partake at specific times of the day or to use particular techniques for preparation or administration.

Injection equipment (needle and syringe) is usually referred to at street level as 'works' and the process of injection is termed 'main-lining', taking a 'fix' or 'shooting-up'. The typical sites chosen for injection are the veins of the forearms, but users may switch to the lower leg, back of the hand, groin or neck if forearm veins are difficult to access. If intravenous access is severely restricted (as may occur in chronic users due to venous damage), the subcutaneous route may be employed. Anabolic steroid users administer their drugs intramuscularly.

The dangers arising from the process of injecting street drugs are discussed below.

INFECTION

Injections of street drugs are usually prepared by dissolving a non-sterile powder or crushed tablet in tap water. This is illustrated in Figure 2.1. Occasionally other liquids are used as diluents, such as lemon juice or vinegar, but this is unusual. The preparation may be heated on an old metal spoon or bottle cap to encourage the drug to enter solution. Some injection drug users may employ citric acid or acetic acid to aid disso-lution of substances such as heroin. Oral liquid preparations such as methadone mixture can also be injected, but may need to be diluted first. Once a solution has been prepared, a filter may then be used to remove any solid particles – commonly this is a cigarette filter, a piece of permeable fabric, cotton wool or blotting paper.

Finally the preparation is injected with a needle and syringe through the skin which is a common source of pathogenic bacteria, especially given the poor personal hygiene of some users. Bacteria on the skin may be carried through it into the bloodstream. The injection equipment may be shared with another or used by the same individual on numerous occasions and may or may not be washed between injec-tions. Even if washing does take place it is frequently done in a manner which does little to prevent contamination.

All of these steps in the injection process are clearly a potential source of contamination with pathogenic organisms – bacteria, viruses and fungi. By conveying a contaminated solution directly into the blood-stream, the individual bypasses all of the body's normal safeguards against the entry of micro-organisms. For this reason, the infections seen

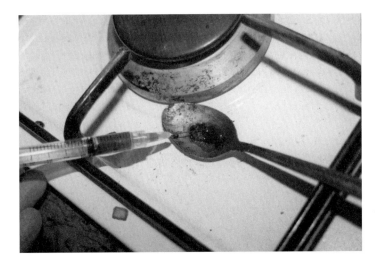

Figure 2.1 The preparation of powdered street drugs for injection involves heating the powder with water to encourage dissolution.

in intravenous drug abusers are frequently well-known conditions but with atypical pathogens, or they may occur in unusual body locations. The likelihood of infection occurring, and of atypical organisms being responsible for them, is further increased if the individual is also suffering immunodeficiency due to AIDS.

Infections can be difficult to diagnose, because of the wide range of micro-organisms which are potentially responsible. However, not all fevers or infections in injection drug users are due to injecting contaminated drug solutions. Many (but by no means all) users have generally poor health due to inadequate nutrition, unsuitable living conditions and deficient personal hygiene, amongst other considerations. In this environment, certain infections are likely to be more common anyway – e.g. chest infections, 'coughs and colds' and urinary tract infections. Tuberculosis and other contagious infections can develop due to association with other sufferers, whether the individual has AIDS or not. Another important point is that withdrawal from some drugs, most notably opioids, can cause fever without any underlying infection.

Attempts at harm reduction have aimed at supplying clean equipment and educating users to try and minimise the risk of infection. Needle and syringe exchange schemes seek to prevent users sharing injection equipment or using the same equipment more than once themselves. The Royal Pharmaceutical Society has prepared guidelines for the establishment of needle exchange schemes and these are reproduced in Appendix A. Users should also be encouraged to clean the injection site immediately before injection to decrease the likelihood of skin commensal contamination. Some organisations suggest that if needles and syringes must be reused, then bleach should be employed as a disinfectant. Users should be constantly encouraged not to share needles and syringes.

Skin and injection site infections

The risk of causing superficial infections is increased when injections are given without cleaning the surface of the skin first. The risk is further increased when injection occurs through parts of the skin that carry a particularly high population of commensal bacteria (e.g. groin) and when injections are deliberately given subcutaneously. Nonetheless skin abscesses are common by most injection routes. Other skin infections that have been reported include cellulitis, necrotising fasciitis, gangrene, septic thrombophlebitis and lymphoedema [1]. The bacteria most commonly involved are *Staphylococcus aureus*, reflecting their prevalence on the surface of the skin itself. *Streptococcus* spp. are probably the next most common, followed by various Gram-negative rods and anaerobic cocci. These skin infections can metastasise to other areas (e.g. bone, heart valves).

Endocarditis

More than half of the intravenous drug abusers presenting with this condition are found to have *Staphylococcus aureus* endocarditis. It is assumed that this organism is derived largely from skin infections. Most infections are thought to be of the tricuspid valve, as after intravenous injection any blood contaminated with micro-organisms will drain into the right side of the heart. However, *Streptococcus* spp. and fungal micro-organisms (especially *Candida* spp.) are more likely to be responsible if the endocarditis affects the left-hand side of the heart. It has been suggested that adulterants in injected drugs, such as starch or lactose, may cause initial damage to the endothelium of the heart. This could then act as a focus for the adherence of platelets and then micro-organisms [2].

Additional organisms which have caused endocarditis in intravenous drug users include other *Staphylococcus* species, *Pseudomonas* spp., *Serratia*, respiratory organisms and anaerobes. One review highlighted how one micro-organism can predominate in a specific geographical location [1]. This is most often linked to the fact that non-staphylococcal endocarditis is likely to be caused by contaminants of the drug itself.

Infective endocarditis responds favourably to antibiotics once the causative organism has been identified. However, long courses of antibiotics (four to six weeks) are often needed.

Viral infection

When injecting street drugs, it is widescale practice to pull on the plunger of the syringe during injection to check that the needle has entered a vein. This results in blood being drawn into the syringe together with any micro-organisms. If the injection equipment is then shared, the second user will inject any pathogenic organisms directly into his or her bloodstream. This has been an important transmission route for the spread of HIV and hepatitis B and C. However, the tip of the needle is contaminated whether or not the individual actually draws blood into the barrel of the syringe, hence users of intramuscular anabolic steroids are also liable to contaminate injection equipment. A full discussion of the implications of HIV status is outside the scope of this book, but those who become immunocompromised as a result of their HIV status are more prone to a whole range of other infections, some of which are diagnostic for AIDS – e.g. *Pneumocystis carinii* pneumonia.

Fungal infections

One review has estimated that fungal infections represent 5 to 50 per cent of serious infections in intravenous drug users [3]. *Candida* spp. are most commonly involved, causing disseminated candidiasis, endo-carditis, central nervous system infections and endophthalmitis. In the 1980s an outbreak of severe *Candida* infections in Europe was found to have arisen because of the use of lemon juice to dissolve heroin prior to injection. This is a known growth medium for fungi [1]. Aspergillosis and mucormycosis have also been described in the injecting population.

Bacterial septicaemia

This can occur, usually secondary to a skin infection. *Streptococcus* spp. are typically responsible. Tetanus has been rarely encountered since the widescale adoption of prophylactic vaccination.

Joint and bone infections

Septic arthritis and osteomyelitis have been described in intravenous drug users. In 1987 a study of 37 heroin abusers with septic arthritis revealed that the joints involved were somewhat atypical. In 16 patients sternoclavicular or sternochondral joints were affected and in 14, sacroiliac joints [4].

IRRITANT EFFECTS

Most drugs that are injected are not themselves irritant. Temazepam and dextropropoxyphene are notable exceptions [5, 6]. They both cause irritation of tissues or veins after injection, leading to abscesses, tissue necrosis, venous fibrosis and phlebitis [7]. These areas of damaged tissue can then act as foci for infection or thrombosis. Irritant effects of most other injectable preparations are largely attributed to adulterants or additives. For example, heroin is often deliberately mixed with acidic substances such as citric acid to aid dissolution. It has also been reported that ammonia may contaminate 'crack' cocaine as a result of the manufacturing procedure. This can be very caustic if injected [8]. Other potentially irritant adulterants in street drugs include quinine and sodium bicarbonate. Clearly irritant effects are more likely to occur if the offending preparation is administered subcutaneously [9] or if there is extravasation during venous injection. Those who inject cocaine may be at particular risk because this drug has local anaesthetic properties which can mask the pain of impending damage.

The repeated intravenous administration of injections at the same location eventually destroys the normal pliable nature of the vein due to the accumulated effects of fibrosis around numerous puncture marks, episodes of phlebitis, infection and the actions of impurities. This requires injection drug users to seek alternative intravenous access sites and eventually, sometimes, to use subcutaneous injection.

EMBOLI, BLOOD VESSEL OCCLUSION AND THROMBOSIS

Most injections given at street level are prepared by mixing a heavily adulterated powder, or a crushed tablet, with water. Most users attempt primitive filtration to try and remove non-soluble particles such as talc, starch and chalk with varying degrees of success. Those that are not removed, or arise from the filter itself, will become microemboli in the bloodstream. In some cases the drug itself may form microemboli (e.g. temazepam [6]). When injected intravenously, these particles can form granulomas in the lung which may impair gaseous diffusion across alveoli (pulmonary granulomatosus) giving rise to dyspnoea, hypoxia, pulmonary hypertension or emphysema. In those who inject stimulants, pulmonary function tests can reveal an obstructive or restrictive pattern [7].

Embolisation of insoluble particles can also cause retinopathy. This has been particularly reported in those injecting crushed methylphenidate tablets, but other crushed tablets and heroin have also been cited as potential causes. In many cases visual acuity is not affected despite the obvious accumulation of obstructive particles in retinal blood vessels. However, impairment of sight can occur. In one study, five out of 23 patients with retinopathy had reduced visual acuity [10].

Occlusion of the small vessels of the retina and lungs can be relatively easy to observe. Embolisation to other parts of the body also occurs but is frequently undetected because it is asymptomatic. In many cases particulate emboli probably dissolve over a period of time leaving no trace. Occlusion of large blood vessels after intravenous injection does not occur as a direct result of particulate contamination but as a consequence of drug-induced phlebitis (see above). This can trigger thrombus formation local to the site of inflammation and subsequently thromboembolism may also occur. Deep vein thromboses are reported quite commonly in the injecting population. However, the most serious forms of blood vessel occlusion occur after intra-arterial injection.

Intra-arterial injection of the contents of temazepam 'gel' capsules has been widely reported as it can result in severe damage to many parts of the body. Often the femoral artery is involved; the patient having mistaken it for the femoral vein. The gel may solidify in blood vessels after injection causing ischaemia and/or act as a focus for thrombus formation by causing an initial damage to the arterial wall (e.g. vasculitis). Temazepam itself is very insoluble and solid particles of it may cause vascular blockade via microembolism [6]; the common practice of filtration through a cigarette filter may also introduce potential microemboli. Severe rhabdomyolysis has been described, necessitating fasciotomy or limb amputation and causing renal failure [11–13]. Other effects which have been reported include deep vein thrombosis (DVT), pulmonary embolus (PE) and critical ischaemia of digits leading to amputation [7, 11, 13–16].

The injection of temazepam gel from capsules represents an extreme example of the potential consequences of intra-arterial injection of irritant substances containing solid particles. Similar effects have been reported after intra-arterial administration of most other parenteral street drugs [17–21]. The general symptoms are swelling distal to the injection site, pain, discolouration, and sensory and/or motor deficit. The subsequent pattern of events will depend on the site of injection and the tissues affected. Muscle ischaemia will cause rhabdomyolysis and its sequelae. Vasculitis is common and this can result in thrombosis of digits leading to gangrene; vasculitis can also trigger thromboembolism which may manifest as DVT or PE. Arterial penetration also increases the risk of serious haemorrhage.

Judging from the number of cases reported in the medical literature, injection of crushed tablets seems to pose a higher risk to the individual than injection of drugs supplied in powder form; temazepam gel appears to pose the highest risk of all.

Air embolus is a potential hazard when large volumes are injected intravenously. A substantial amount of air in the heart causes blood to froth in the chambers during pumping leading to inefficiency and heart failure. It has been estimated that 10 ml of air would be required in the heart to cause failure [22]; this would be very difficult to achieve after injection with a hand-held syringe and is unlikely to occur at street level.

PHARMACOLOGICAL EFFECTS

Compared to oral administration, the pharmacological effects of street drugs appear much more rapidly after intravenous injection. The effects may in some cases also be more dramatic. Large doses of intravenous opioids are known to cause sudden respiratory depression and death. Usually this occurs because a sample of heroin is more potent than the user anticipated. However, fentanyl analogues are particularly powerful drugs which are known to have caused death so rapidly that individuals have died with the needle still in place (see Chapter 3).

One reasonably common reaction that can occur after intravenous administration of most street drugs is fainting. In one study of 13 methylphenidate abusers, 12 reported fainting immediately after injection [23]; in a study of 23 temazepam abusers, 12 reported 'blackouts' after injection [7].

Adulterants

At street level no drugs are pure. A variety of cheap inert or pharmacologically active adulterants are used to dilute the drug. The active adulterants are often those considered appropriate to the illicit drug in question. For example, amphetamine, cocaine and ecstasy may be contaminated with stimulants such as other amphetamine derivatives, pseudoephedrine and caffeine. Ecstasy can be cut with ketamine or other drugs with broadly similar effects (see Chapter 6). Cocaine may be adulterated with local anaesthetics [24]. The pharmacological effects of contaminants or adulterants may be important. Thrombocytopenia has been reported in intravenous heroin users and is believed to be an immune reaction to an unknown toxin [25, 26]. Thrombocytopenia explicitly caused by quinine in street drugs has been identified [27]. Quinine can also be a venous irritant. Two deaths associated with strychnine contamination of street drugs have also been described [28]. Strychnine can be found in heroin or cocaine. Arsenic can be a common adulterant of opium in some areas [29].

'STIGMATA'

Repeated intravenous injection over a prolonged period frequently results in certain characteristic changes around veins which mark the individual as an intravenous drug user. These are most frequently seen in the forearm. These may include needle marks, scarring due to abscesses, bruising, and discolouration of the skin along the line of veins due to insoluble particles accumulating within the skin.

REFERENCES

1. Cherubin, C.E. and Sapira, J.D. (1993) The medical complications of drug addiction and the medical assessment of the intravenous drug user: 25 years later. *Ann. Intern. Med.* **119**: 1017–1028.
2. Gribbin, R.B. and Crook, D.W.M. (1996) Infective endocarditis, in *Oxford Textbook of Medicine*, Oxford University Press, Oxford, pp. 2436–2451.
3. Leen, C.L.S. and Brettle, R.P. (1991) Fungal infections in drug users. *J. Antimicrob. Chemother.* **28(A)**: 83–96.
4. Lopez-Longo, F.J., Menard, H.A., Carreno, L. *et al.* (1987) Primary septic arthritis in heroin users: early diagnosis by radioisotopic imaging and geographic variations in the causative agents. *J. Rheumatol.* **14**: 991–994.
5. Tennant, F.S. (1973) Complications of propoxyphene abuse. *Arch. Intern. Med.* **132**: 191–194.
6. Launchbury, A.P., Drake, J. and Seager, H. (1992) Misuse of temazepam (letter); *Br. Med. J.* **305**: 252–253.
7. Ruben, S.M. and Morrison, C.L. (1992) Temazepam misuse in a group of injecting drug users. *Br. J. Addiction,* **87**: 1387–1392.
8. Pickering, H., Donoghoe, M., Green, A. and Foster, R. (1993) Crack injection. *Druglink,* **8**: 12.
9. Thomas III, W.O., Almand, J.D., Stark, G.B., Parry, S.W. and Rodning, C.B. (1995) Hand injuries secondary to subcutaneous illicit drug injections. *Ann. Plastic Surg.* **34**: 27–31.
10. Tse, D.T. and Ober, R.R. (1980) Talc retinopathy. *Am. J. Ophthalmol.* **90**: 624–640.
11. Scott, R.N., Woodburn, K.R., Reid, D.B., *et al.* (1992) Intra-arterial temazepam (letter). *Br. Med. J.* **304**: 1630.
12. Adiseshiah, M., Jones, D.A. and Round, J.M. (1992) Intra-arterial temazepam (letter) *Br. Med. J.* **304**: 1630.
13. Blair, S.D., Holcombe, C., Coombes, E.N. and O'Malley, M.K. (1991) Leg ischaemia secondary to non-medical injection of temazepam (letter). *Lancet,* **338**: 1393–1394.
14. Fox, R., Beeching, N.J., Morrison, C., Ruben, S. and Garvey, T.(1991) Leg ischaemia secondary to non-medical injection of temazepam (letter). *Lancet,* **338**: 253.

15. Dodd, T.J., Scott, R.N., Woodburn, K.R. and Going, T.J. (1994) Limb ischaemia after intra-arterial injection of temazepam gel: histology of nine cases. *J. Clin. Pathol.* **47**: 512–514.

16. Vella, E.J. and Edwards, C.W. (1993) Death from pulmonary microembolisation after intravenous injection of temazepam. *Br. Med. J.* **307**: 26.

17. Om, A., Ellahham, S. and DiSciascio, G. (1993) Management of cocaine-induced cardiovascular complications. *Am. Heart J.* **125**: 469–475.

18. Begg, E.J., McGrath, M.A. and Wade, D.N. (1980) Inadvertent intra-arterial injection. *Med. J. Aust.* **2**: 561–563.

19. Borrero, E. (1995) Treatment of 'trash hand' following intra-arterial injection of drugs in addicts – case studies. *Vasc. Surg.* **29**: 71–75.

20. Stueber, K. (1987) The treatment of intra-arterial pentazocine injection injuries with intra-arterial reserpine. *Ann. Plastic Surg.* **18**: 41–46.

21. Samuel, I., Bishop, C.C.R. and Jamieson, C.W. (1993) Accidental intra-arterial drug injection successfully treated with Iloprost. *Eur. J. Vasc. Surg.* **7**: 93–94.

22. Gunson, H.H. and Martlew, V.J. (1996) Blood replacement, in *Oxford Textbook of Medicine*, Oxford University Press, Oxford, pp. 3687–3696.

23. Parran, T.V. and Jasinski, D.R. (1991) Intravenous methylphenidate abuse – prototype for prescription drug abuse. *Arch. Intern. Med.* **151**: 781–783.

24. Shannon, M. (1988) Clinical toxicity of cocaine adulterants. *Ann. Emerg. Med.* **17**: 1243–1247.

25. Adams, W.H., Rufo, R.A., Talarico, L., Silverman, S.L. and Brauer, M.J. (1978) Thrombocytopenia and intravenous heroin use. *Ann. Intern. Med.* **89**: 207–211.

26. Warkenstein, T.E. (1994) Thrombocytopenia and illicit drug use (letter). *Ann. Intern. Med.* **120**: 693.

27. Christie, D.J., Walker, R.H., Kolins, M.D., Wilner, F.M. and Aster, R.H. (1983) Quinine-induced thrombocytopenia following intravenous use of heroin. *Ann. Intern. Med.* **143**: 1174–1175.

28. Decker, W.J., Baker, H.E., Tamulinas, S.H. and Korndorffer, W.E. (1982) Two deaths resulting from apparent parenteral injection of strychnine. *Vet. Hum. Toxicol.* **24**: 161–162.

29. Wijesekera, A.R.L., Henry, K.D. and Ranasighe, P. (1988) The detection and estimation of (A) arsenic in opium, and (B) strychnine in opium and heroin, as a means of identification of their respective sources. *Forensic Sci. Int.* **36**: 193–209.

3

Opioids

If opium-eating be a sensual pleasure, and if I am bound to confess that I have indulged in it to an excess not yet recorded of any other man, it is no less true that I have struggled against this fascination with a fervent zeal, and have at length accomplished what I never yet heard attributed to any other man, have untwisted, almost to its final links, the chain which fettered me.

Thomas de Quincy, 'Confessions of an English Opium Eater', 1821.

HISTORY

Opiates were originally available from the opium poppy (*Papaver somniferum*), native to Asia Minor (Figure 3.1). The active constituents can be found in the latex which exudes from incisions in the unripe capsule of the flowering head. The alkaloids which occur in the poppy include morphine, noscapine, codeine, papaverine and thebaine. Strictly speaking, alkaloids derived from the opium poppy which have morphine-like actions are termed opiates, whereas opioids are synthetic derivatives, e.g. methadone. However, in recent times the term opioid has been understood to encompass opiates.

Morphine is responsible for most of the psychotropic activity and comprises some 9 to 17 per cent of the weight of dried opium but is usually about 10 per cent. Opium itself has been used by man for thousands of years, both as a medicine and as an intoxicant. It was cultivated in many places in Neolithic Europe, where it may have been burned to produce an intoxicating smoke. However, in most cultures, opium was usually taken orally. Smoking of opium using an individual pipe probably originated in China in the 17th century and a huge population of

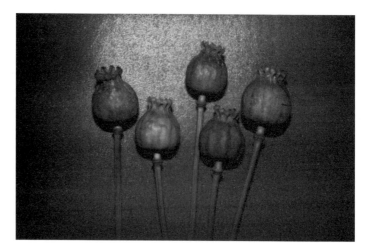

Figure 3.1 Heads of opium poppies.

dependent individuals began to develop there. Opium was subsequently the cause of two wars between Britain and China in the 19th century when the British continued to sell opium to the Chinese people despite a decree from the Emperor outlawing the use of it.

In the USA, the widescale use of opium as an analgesic during the Civil War created many thousands of addicts. In both the USA and Great Britain opium purchased for 'medicinal purposes' and sold overtly to produce intoxication caused serious social problems in the 19th century. Many medicines that were freely sold over the counter for coughs, gastrointestinal complaints, sleep disorders etc. contained appreciable quantities of opium. The extent of this problem was not recognised for many years; it abated to some extent following legislation. The problem of opioid abuse has remained ever since, in one form or another. Today, most abuse is centred around heroin (diamorphine).

Morphine was first isolated in 1806 by a pharmacist, Wilhelm Sertürner, and named after the Greek god of dreams, Morpheus. Like many products since, diamorphine was initially marketed (in 1898) as a 'less addictive' form of an existing drug and only later was its true dependence potential realised.

EFFECTS SOUGHT

When heroin is injected the user commonly experiences a rapid feeling of intense pleasure. This euphoria is replaced by a feeling of warmth (resulting from peripheral vasodilation), relaxation and happiness – although some experience stimulatory effects. Unlike a variety of other central nervous system (CNS) depressants, doses sufficient to cause euphoria do not impair movement (ataxia) or intellectual ability. Large doses produce sedation or a pleasant light sleep. The individual is able to detach himself from the ongoing concerns and pressures of real life. With chronic administration, however, the addict becomes tolerant to the psychotropic effects which were the original purpose of abuse. The object of each 'fix' then effectively becomes to avoid withdrawal symptoms (negative reinforcement).

Smoking, vaporising or 'snorting' heroin produces a milder 'rush' than intravenous injection. The oral route does not produce a 'rush' and is therefore unpopular. Non-heroin opioids produce similar but usually less intense effects, because of reduced CNS penetration and potency. The fentanyl derivatives are a notable exception.

ADMINISTRATION

Probably all of the opioids available medicinally have been abused to some extent. The heroin abused on the street today is made illegally in small-scale laboratories in the UK and abroad, and very little is diverted from legitimate medical sources. However, supplies of most other opioids are largely obtained through abuse of pharmaceutical products, e.g. methadone, buprenorphine, Diconal and dextropropoxyphene.

Heroin is the most widely used opioid, probably because of its potency, solubility in water and high biological lipophilicity, which affords rapid brain access. It is known as 'junk', 'H', 'smack', 'skag' or 'horse'. It is usually supplied as a brown or off-white powder, depending on the purity and the manufacturing process. It is always adulterated with other substances when bought at street level. The drug is progressively diluted (or 'cut') as it moves down the line from manufacturer through various dealers to the end user. Adulterants include almost any powder, e.g. sugars, talcum powder, chalk, flour, salt and other drugs. A typical dealer's preparation slab is shown in Figure 3.2.

Diconal has a certain appeal because it contains an opioid, dipipanone, as well as cyclizine. The abuse potential of this antihistamine is discussed in Chapter 12.

Buprenorphine, a partial opioid agonist, was initially claimed to have low dependency potential and to produce only mild symptoms upon withdrawal. However, perhaps predictably, buprenorphine abuse eventually became so widespread in the UK that it forced the reclassification of this drug from prescription-only to controlled drug.

Dextropropoxyphene, dihydrocodeine and codeine are less popular at street level because they are weak opioids and because many

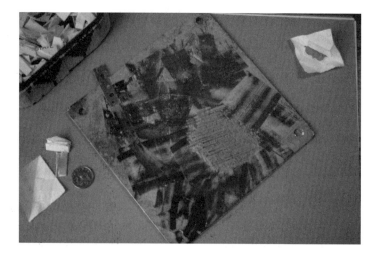

Figure 3.2 A heroin dealer's slab. Powdered heroin is 'cut' with an inert powder on a smooth surface, such as a mirror, using a razor blade. Resultant powders are sold in small bags or card 'wraps' as here.

pharmaceutical sources containing a sufficient amount of opioid also contain paracetamol or aspirin. Consequently, it is difficult to take enough of the opioid for intoxication without risking potentially fatal paracetamol/aspirin overdose. An exception to this is codeine linctus but it has the disadvantage to the abuser of a low concentration, such that the large volume required for intoxication prevents injection. Dextropropoxyphene, dihydrocodeine and codeine are weak opioids and only likely to be taken when more potent alternatives are not available, so that illicit synthesis is unlikely to be profitable. Nonetheless, these opioids are still abused, particularly codeine linctus. The abuse of over-the-counter opioids is discussed in more detail in Chapter 12.

The methadone encountered at street level has been diverted from treatment clinics where the drug is prescribed as a substitute for street opioids in dependent individuals (see below). In the USA, illicit derivatives of fentanyl, a very potent opioid, have gained in popularity but these are not widely used in the UK (see below).

Most of the opioids can be administered orally, but the CNS effects are slow to develop and are blunted. In addition, all opioids are subject to some presystemic metabolism – the average bioavailability of oral buprenorphine is only 16 per cent, for example, whereas for morphine it is 40 to 50 per cent. Many addicts prefer the intravenous route as this produces an intense 'rush' of euphoria which does not occur following oral ingestion. A variety of unsuitable preparations are injected (or 'fixed'), including heroin powder bought on the street, crushed opioid-containing tablets and liquid preparations (e.g. methadone elixir). For the purpose of injecting, street heroin is sometimes mixed by the abuser with simple organic acids (e.g. ascorbic acid, citric acid) to facilitate extraction of heroin from the mixture of inactive adulterants; occasionally lemon juice or vinegar is used. Persistent injection of non-sterile solutions which are contaminated with particles eventually causes blood vessel damage, which, in turn, severely restricts venous access (see Chapter 2). If this occurs, addicts may sometimes resort to subcutaneous injection.

Powdered heroin can be inhaled nasally ('snorted'), smoked in cigarettes ('reefers') or heated on foil and the vapour inhaled ('chasing the dragon' or 'skagging'). Non-injection forms of administration are becoming more common, particularly in new and younger heroin users. This is probably related to the fact that heroin supplies have become more pure in the past decade, enabling addicts to 'snort' or 'chase the dragon' and produce an acceptable 'rush' without the risk of infection inherent in intravenous injection [1, 2]. This reduces the risk of AIDS due to shared injection equipment. It remains to be seen whether these novices will in time move towards injecting.

PHARMACOKINETICS AND PHARMACOLOGY

Opioid receptors in the central nervous system mediate the actions of endogenous peptides such as enkephalins and dynorphins, which probably initiate or control a range of behaviours and moods. There may be up to five types of receptor: μ (mu), κ (kappa), σ (sigma), δ (delta) and ε (epsilon). The euphoria and physical dependence attributable to opioids are thought to be mediated through μ receptors. Receptors outside the CNS facilitate some of the peripheral side effects of opioids, e.g. constipation and effects on renal blood flow.

The opioids are all metabolised principally in the liver and the metabolites are then excreted renally. Diamorphine (heroin) is unusual in that the molecule itself has no intrinsic actions at opioid receptors, all of its actions are due to its two main metabolites: 6-monoacetyl-morphine and morphine. Diamorphine (or diacetylmorphine) is rapidly deacetylated in the liver, kidney, blood, brain and other tissues to form these metabolites, such that diamorphine has an average half-life of only three minutes; 6-monoacetylmorphine has a similarly short half-life. Morphine is converted to a range of metabolites in the liver and has an average half-life of about three hours. The two most important metabolites are formed by conjugation: morphine-3-glucuronide and morphine-6-glucuronide. The latter only compromises about 5 per cent of metabolites, but is a much more potent opioid agonist than morphine. All the morphine metabolites are excreted renally.

ADVERSE EFFECTS

The adverse effects associated with opioid abuse fall into four distinct categories: side effects of opioid drugs, effects of overdose, adverse consequences of the abuse process and withdrawal symptoms.

The side effects of opioids are well-known and are listed in Table 3.1. Tolerance develops to all of these dose-related effects except constipation. Thrombocytopenia has been reported, but may be an immune-based reaction to adulterants [3]. Chronic administration tends to depress sexual desire and performance, although these may be enhanced in the initial stages of abuse.

Intoxication with opioids may increase the chance of the individual causing or being exposed to accidents. Disinhibition and subjectively enhanced sexual performance (especially in the early stages of heroin use) can result in increased sexual activity and therefore increased risk of AIDS, other sexually-transmitted diseases or unwanted pregnancies.

The effects of overdose are given in Table 3.2. All of these, except arrhythmia and pulmonary oedema, may be reversed with the opioid antagonist naloxone, but at the risk of precipitating acute opioid withdrawal. The dose of naloxone needs to be repeated because it has

Table 3.1 Adverse effects of opioids

Common
- Nausea, vomiting, constipation
- Drowsiness, mental confusion

Infrequent
- Sweating, facial flushing, pruritus
- Dry mouth
- Hallucinations, dysphoria
- Urinary retention
- Headache

Rare
- Thrombocytopenia
- Rashes, urticaria
- Vertigo
- Palpitations, postural hypotension

Table 3.2 Signs and symptoms of opioid overdose

- Dysphoria, hallucinations, heavy sedation
- Miosis
- Hypothermia
- Respiratory depression, pulmonary oedema, coma
- Hypotension, bradycardia, arrhythmias secondary to hypoxia
- Convulsions (dextropropoxyphene and pethidine only)

a shorter half-life than most opioids. Some drugs, such as dextro-propoxyphene, methadone and buprenorphine, have particularly long half-lives and prolonged naloxone administration may therefore be required after overdose with these substances (up to 72 hours with methadone). Opioid overdose may occur with the intention of committing suicide. But it may arise by accident as a result of the unexpected potency of a sample purchased at street level or after a period of abstinence during which tolerance has decreased. The incidence of overdose amongst heroin users has been estimated at about one-quarter of the affected population in a London study [4], but two-thirds of the population in Sydney, Australia [5]. Consequently it has recently been proposed that the opioid antagonist naloxone be supplied to street users of opioids [6].

Adverse effects arising from the abuse process include the harmful consequences of injection, which are discussed in Chapter 2. There are also a large number of adverse social effects which result from opioid dependence, including increased likelihood of criminal activity, general poor health and diet, antisocial behaviour and disrupted relationships.

OPIOID DEPENDENCE

Opioid dependence is a well-established and clearly defined phenomenon. It is characterised by physical dependence which becomes more likely as the dose and duration of administration increase. There are two essential components to this: receptor tolerance and a withdrawal reaction upon discontinuation.

Opioid addicts become tolerant to the pleasurable psychotropic effects quite rapidly. The dose is increased in an attempt to regain the lost experience. This is effective for a time, but tolerance redevelops and the dose is then progressively increased to a maximum, often determined by drug availability. At this level there is permanent tolerance to most of the effects of opioids, including euphoria, although complete tolerance to constipation and miosis does not seem to occur. The drive to continue drug administration becomes the desire to avoid a with-drawal reaction (negative reinforcement) rather than the pleasure of the experience (positive reinforcement). Cross-tolerance exists between all the opioid drugs and so addicts may seek cheaper alternatives to street opioids in an attempt to stave off withdrawal when these are not available. Codeine linctus in particular is used for this purpose.

The opioid withdrawal syndrome is characterised by a range of symptoms (see Table 3.3). When an addict attempts to cease opioid administration abruptly, without medical support, he or she is said to be doing 'cold turkey'. This is believed to originate from the gooseflesh appearance of the skin that is commonly seen in this situation. The symptoms of withdrawal manifest as the reverse of normal opioid action on the body, i.e. they are suggestive of CNS hyperactivity rather than depression. Although subjectively very unpleasant, these effects are not life-threatening, and the subject remains relatively lucid throughout.

Signs of heroin withdrawal may commence within six hours of abstinence, but the peak effects are seen after 36 to 72 hours, followed by gradual abatement over the subsequent 5 to 10 days. If opioid addicts are given naloxone, withdrawal may develop almost instantly.

This acute phase of withdrawal is followed by a period of relatively chronic symptoms usually characterised by a craving for opioids and accompanied by anxiety, emotional lability, depression, fatigue or

Table 3.3 Symptoms of acute opioid withdrawal

Initial symptoms
- Anxiety, restlessness, insomnia
- Mild tachypnoea, yawning, coughing, sneezing
- Craving for drug
- Lacrimation, perspiration, rhinorrhoea

Later symptoms
- Tremors, myalgia, arthralgia, muscle twitching
- Chills, piloerection (gooseflesh), hot flushes
- Anorexia, abdominal pains
- Mydriasis
- Insomnia, headache

Severe cases
- Tachycardia, hypertension or hypotension
- Nausea, vomiting, diarrhoea
- Fever, dehydration
- Severe or persistent tachypnoea
- Agitation

insomnia. These persistent effects can take months to abate, are very hard to ignore and may encourage a return to opioid abuse.

Recent work in animals has helped to elucidate the mechanisms of opioid withdrawal. The locus coeruleus in the brain seems to play a particularly important part in mediating the physical signs of opioid withdrawal. Furthermore, the existence of anti-opioid peptides has been postulated [7]. These peptides may be released in the CNS as a response to chronic exogenous opioid administration and therefore help to mediate tolerance. The excess anti-opioid peptides that remain following opioid discontinuation may at least be partly responsible for causing the symptoms of withdrawal.

Treatment of dependence and withdrawal

Opioid dependence should not be seen as a hopeless cause. A 22-year follow-up of 128 heroin injectors from London in 1996, revealed that 50 per cent of them had stopped using opioids [8] (this included seven non-users who had died from natural causes unrelated to addiction). Opioid addicts seeking assistance should be referred to drug dependence treatment units (DDUs) where staff are trained to deal with the problem and psychiatrists are licensed by the Home Office to prescribe the required treatment. The immediate aim of attending such a clinic is not necessarily withdrawal from opioids, but this can be achieved in one of three ways.

1. without any support medication ('cold turkey');
2. with support medication;
3. by substitution of another opioid for the abused substance and withdrawing this slowly.

Unsupported withdrawal usually only occurs when addicts decide to stop on their own initiative or if supplies of opioid are interrupted for any length of time, so forcing the addict into withdrawal (e.g. imprisonment, hospitalisation). The Department of Health recommends a variety of drugs that may provide symptomatic relief of some of the effects of withdrawal. These include propranolol, thioridazine and even benzodiazepines [9]. However, a short course of clonidine is particularly useful for suppressing the signs of acute opioid withdrawal, although it does not prevent the more chronic symptoms which develop after the acute phase. Overactivity of central adrenergic neurones is thought to mediate many of the effects of withdrawal and this activity is suppressed by clonidine [10], a presynaptic alpha-2 adrenergic agonist which inhibits neurotransmitter release. Side effects may include sedation, dry mouth and hypotension. The latter side-effect makes it wise to monitor the patient after the first few doses. Clonidine is not licensed for this purpose, although the similar drug lofexidine is. Data on the efficacy of lofexidine are largely derived from open trials and no comparative studies involving the more widely used clonidine have been published. Lofexidine although effective is also more expensive than clonidine. Other alpha-2 adrenergic agonists which have been investigated include guanabenz and guanfacine. None of these drugs reduce craving for opioids, which is the most significant cause of recidivism.

A substitute opioid can be prescribed to addicts in a dose sufficient to prevent withdrawal symptoms with one of two objectives. Prescribing daily maintenance doses may allow addicts to lead comparatively normal lives unperturbed by cravings for heroin, drug-seeking behaviour and all the concomitant unhealthy aspects of the street addict's lifestyle. Some addicts may receive daily maintenance doses of medication indefinitely. Alternatively, the substitute may offer a convenient 'bridge' between an old drug culture lifestyle and the prospect of a drug-free existence. Once stabilised upon a suitable dose, patients can begin a structured withdrawal programme, involving gradual dosage reduction over weeks.

The substitute opioid most commonly used is methadone, usually as the elixir (1 mg/ml), but intravenous methadone can be made available for the few patients that find it difficult to abandon the injection habit. However, injection should be the exception rather than the rule and the number of prescriptions for methadone injection (estimated at over 9 per cent of the total) has been criticised [11]. If the dose of opioid abused is known, a dose of methadone of equivalent potency can be given [9]. If the dose is not known, and for street heroin this is invariably the case, methadone must be titrated to symptoms of withdrawal. Methadone has a long half-life, allowing once daily administration when used chronically although more frequent administration may be needed initially.

Another advantage of the long half-life is that although withdrawal symptoms tend to be more sustained than those associated with heroin, they are also milder; clonidine or lofexidine can be useful to further reduce severity. Signs of methadone withdrawal begin about 36–72 hours after the last dose or dosage reduction. The duration of the withdrawal programme is highly variable and is best individualised according to the subject's response and circumstances. It is probably better to reduce the dosage quickly in the early stages, followed by a more prolonged series of reductions later [9]. As mentioned above, complete detoxification may not be appropriate or desirable for all addicts.

It is important to realise that supply of methadone itself is not all that is required. If true social rehabilitation is to occur, full counselling and psychosocial support is necessary to prevent a return to old habits. Some addicts may use prescribed methadone to provide a baseline plasma level on which 'top-ups' of street drugs can be superimposed. Clearly this defeats the object of treatment. It can be identified by random urine tests during clinic visits. Work in the USA suggests that prescribing larger doses of methadone may counteract this problem [12, 13]. Typically, UK methadone maintenance doses are less than 50 mg daily. In the USA, doses of 50 to 100 mg per day are used. These doses are believed to induce such a high level of opioid tolerance that 'top-up' doses of street heroin have no effects. However, in the presence of liver disease, consideration should be given to the use of low doses, as methadone is cleared hepatically. Ten deaths were reported from Australia in 1990 in patients with hepatitis who died within two to six days of starting an average of 60 mg of methadone per day [14]. It is possible that methadone accumulated to toxic levels.

Several clinics in England now supply heroin reefers in addition to, or instead of, oral methadone [15]. These provide the 'rush' that addicts expect and seem to avoid the need for injections of street heroin. The Royal Pharmaceutical Society of Great Britain has developed a protocol giving guidance on the preparation of these reefers [16]. This is reproduced in Appendix B.

Methadone must be supplied with care, because it is clearly a substance that might itself be abused. The drug does appear on the street because addicts may swap their medication for other drugs of abuse or simply sell it. In addition, deaths may occur when non-tolerant individuals ingest this very potent drug [17]. A single 50 to 100 mg dose of methadone can produce life-threatening effects in a new adult user and there have been a number of fatal accidental poisonings reported in the children of opioid-addicted parents.

Individuals maintained on methadone commonly require antidepressants and laxatives as additional medication. It should be noted that recipients of regular maintenance doses of methadone may still genuinely require opioid analgesia. Since they are completely tolerant to the effects of methadone, analgesia should be prescribed in the usual way (i.e. on top of maintenance methadone [18]), with due deference to the potential for abuse and the need to prevent constipation by prescribing laxatives.

Other opioids have been used as maintenance treatment or to aid withdrawal. Most notable among these is levomethadyl acetate (LAAM), a potent opioid with a duration of action of some 72 hours. The long half-life of the parent drug and its metabolites allow administration three times weekly. The US Food and Drug Administration has approved levomethadyl as an alternative to methadone in treatment clinics. Other opioids which have been used include dextropropoxyphene and buprenorphine. The latter agent has partial agonist properties – it will give some rewarding opioid-like CNS effects but it may also antagonise the psychotropic effects of any heroin taken surreptitiously while on a treatment programme.

Naltrexone is an orally active opioid antagonist. Unlike buprenorphine, naltrexone has no agonist effects and antagonises the effect of opioids without the reward of an opioid 'buzz'. This has severely limited the usefulness of the drug but it may be effective in preventing relapse in highly motivated people who have successfully negotiated acute opioid withdrawal because it not only prevents positive reinforcement but may diminish craving.

The experimental drug ibogaine may offer some hope to those dependent upon opioids. It is claimed to halt the craving for opioids which occurs in those who are attempting abstinence [19, 20]. There has been concern over the potential toxicity of ibogaine and some deaths have been reported. At the time of writing the only information on efficacy comes from animal studies and largely anecdotal human experiences. The drug is itself psychoactive and those who use it experience a 24-36 hour 'trip' after one dose. Individuals are purported to emerge from this state free from opioid craving. In an open study of seven patients dependent upon heroin in 1994, three remained drug-free 14 weeks after completion of the study [21].

DESIGNER OPIOIDS

Fentanyl-based designer drugs are rarely seen in the UK but have been widely abused in the USA [22, 23]. As a group, the fentanyl-derived opioids are often sold under the name of 'synthetic heroin'. The most well-known example is alpha-methylfentanyl known on the street as 'China white'; another example is 3-methylfentanyl ('3MF' or 'TMF'). These and other analogues can be over one thousand times more potent than heroin and have a short duration of action (typically 30 to 90 minutes). The two properties combined dramatically increase the positive reinforcement potential and therefore the risk of dependence occurring after only a few doses. They are usually injected but smoking or nasal inhalation is becoming more common. The drugs produce intense opioid effects with a very rapid onset and they can cause dramatic, sudden respiratory depression and death. Many deaths have been reported in the USA – in some cases death was so quick that abusers have been found with the needle still *in situ* [22, 24]. Unfortunately, fentanyl derivatives are not detected by routine immunoassay screening tests for opioids and so may not always be identified [25].

Pethidine analogues have also been reported from the USA – one in particular has come to the attention of the public: 1-methyl-4-phenyl-4-propionoxypiperidine (MPPP). Several batches of illicitly produced MPPP were contaminated with MPTP, a very potent neurotoxin which caused irreversible brain damage with Parkinsonian-like symptoms [22, 24].

REFERENCES

1. Strang, J., Griffiths, P., Powis, B. and Gossop, M. (1992) First use of heroin: changes in route of administration over time. *Br. Med. J.* **304**: 1222–1223.
2. French, J.F. and Safford, J. (1989) AIDS and intranasal heroin (letter). *Lancet*, i: 1082.
3. Adams, W.H., Rufo, R.A., Talarico, L., Silverman, S.L. and Brauer, M.J. (1978) Thrombocytopenia and intravenous heroin use. *Ann. Intern. Med.* **89**: 207–211.
4. Gossop, M., Griffiths, P., Powis, B., Williamson, S. and Strang, J. (1996) Frequency of non-fatal heroin overdose: survey of heroin users recruited in non-clinical settings. *Br. Med. J.* **313**: 402.
5. Darke, S., Ross, J. and Hall, W. (1995) Overdose among heroin users in Sydney, Australia, I. Prevalates and correlates of non-fatal overdose. *Addiction*, **91**: 405–411.
6. Strang, J., Darke, S., Hall, W., Farrell, M. and Ali, R. (1996) Heroin overdose: the case for take-home naloxone. *Br. Med. J.* **312**: 1435–1436.
7. Rothman, R.B. (1992) A review of the role of anti-opioid peptides in morphine tolerance and dependence. *Synapse*, **12**: 129–138.
8. Tobutt, C., Oppenheimer, E. and Laranjeira, R. (1996) Health of cohort of heroin addicts from London clinics: 22 year follow-up. *Br. Med. J.* **312**: 1458.
9. Department of Health (1991) *Drug Misuse and Dependence: Guidelines on Clinical Management.* Report of a medical working group. HMSO, London.
10. Guthrie, S.K. (1990) Pharmacologic interventions for the treatment of opioid dependence and withdrawal. *Ann. Pharmacother.* **24**: 721–734.
11. Strang, J., Sheridan, J. and Barber, N. (1996) Prescribing injectable and oral methadone to opiate addicts: results from the 1995 national postal survey of community pharmacies in England and Wales. *Br. Med. J.* **313**: 270–272.

12. D'Aunno, T. and Vaughn, T.E. (1992) Variations in methadone treatment practices: results from a national study. *J. Am. Med. Assoc.* **267**: 253–258.

13. Cooper, J.R. (1992) Ineffective use of psychoactive drugs – methadone treatment is no exception (editorial). *J. Am. Med. Assoc.* **267**: 281–282.

14. Drummer, O.H., Syrjanen, M., Opeskin, K. and Cordner, S. (1990) Deaths of heroin addicts starting on a methadone maintenance programme (letter). *Lancet,* **335**: 108

15. Marks, J.A. and Palombella, A. (1990) Prescribing smokable drugs (letter). *Lancet,* **335**: 864.

16. Royal Pharmaceutical Society of Great Britain (1994) Heroin reefers – a protocol. *Pharm. J.* **252**: 53–54.

17. Harding-Pink, D. (1993) Opioid toxicity – methadone: one person's maintenance dose is another's poison. *Lancet,* **341**: 665–666.

18. Savage, S.R. (1993) Addiction in the treatment of pain: significance, recognition and management. *J. Pain Symptom Management,* **8**: 265–278.

19. Anon. (1995) Anti-addiction drug ibogaine on trial. *Nat. Med.* **1**: 288–289.

20. Anon. (1993) Ibogaine. *NIDA Capsule (CAP 53)* , National Institute on Drug Abuse, USA, pp. 1–2.

21. Sheppard, S.G. (1994) A preliminary investigation of ibogaine: case reports and recommendations for further study. *J. Substance Abuse Treat,* **11**: 379–385.

22. Anon. (1993) Designer drugs. *NIDA Capsule (CAP10)* , National Institute on Drug Abuse, USA, pp. 1–3.

23. Hibbs, J., Perper, J. and Winek, C.L. (1991) An outbreak of designer drug-related deaths in Pennsylvania. *J. Am. Med. Assoc.* **265**: 1011–1013.

24. Buchanan, J.F. and Brown, C.R. (1988) 'Designer drugs' – a problem in clinical toxicology. *Med. Toxicol.* **3**: 1–17.

25. Berens, A.I.L., Voets, A.J. and Demedts, P. (1996) Illicit fentanyl in Europe (letter). *Lancet,* **347**: 1334–1335.

4

Cannabis

When you return to this mundane sphere from your visionary world, you would seem to leave a Neapolitan spring for a Lapland winter – to quit paradise for earth – heaven for hell! Taste the hashish, guest of mine – taste the hashish!
Alexandre Dumas, 'The Count of Monte Cristo', 1844.

HISTORY

The term 'cannabis' actually refers to a variety of preparations which are derived from the Indian hemp, *Cannabis sativa*. This dioecious, bushy plant was originally native to India, Bangladesh and Pakistan but is now considerably more widely disseminated largely due to the intervention of man. It is illustrated in Figure 4.1. Historically, cannabis has been an important plant with three key properties. First it has been used for thousands of years as a source of fibre for making rope and textiles. Secondly, the seeds are a source of food and of oil for lamps. Finally the resin has been used as a medicine and as an intoxicant.

Cannabis was known to the ancient Chinese at least 5000 years ago and it is mentioned in an Egyptian papyrus dated to 1600 BC. The Greeks and Romans also made use of the cannabis plant. Interestingly, there are no records of these four early civilisations using cannabis intentionally to produce intoxication for pleasure, despite the popularity of alcohol for this purpose. By contrast there is a relatively long tradition of this practice in eastern Europe, India and 'Arabia'. The taking of cannabis for pleasure in western Europe and the USA began in the mid-19th century but only became a widespread practice from the 1960s onwards.

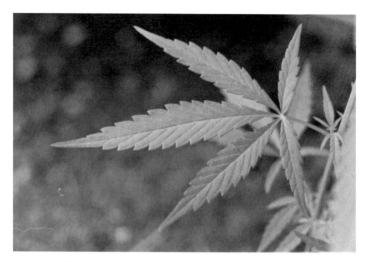

Figure 4.1   The distinctive leaf of *Cannabis sativa*, the Indian hemp.

Glandular hairs (trichomes) which secrete the resin are most abundant in the flowering heads and surrounding leaves. The psychoactive constituents of the resin are termed cannabinoids. There are over 60 of these but the most important psychoactive compound is delta-9-tetrahydrocannabinol (THC). Cannabidiol and cannabinol are other constituents which have been extensively investigated for pharmacological activity. The amount of resin secreted is strongly influenced by weather conditions during growth, the sex of the plant (females produce more) and the time of harvest. Although it is illegal to grow cannabis in the UK without a licence, home-grown illicit production does occur on a small scale. However, unless grown under specially controlled conditions these plants have a low resin yield because of the unsuitability of the British climate.

Cannabis has several potential medical uses (see Table 4.1). Historically the resin has been used to treat a huge variety of inappropriate conditions and many claims have been made for therapeutic efficacy with little or no evidence to support them. Several synthetic cannabinoids have been investigated for therapeutic efficacy, but only nabilone and dronabinol are still used medicinally in the West. Dronabinol is structurally identical to naturally occurring THC.

EFFECTS SOUGHT

Cannabis is the most commonly abused illicit substance in Britain. A Gallup poll in the UK in 1989 reported that 12 per cent of the

Table 4.1   Uses of cannabis or cannabinoids

Established uses
- Chemotherapy-induced nausea and vomiting (e.g. nabilone, dronabinol)
- Appetite stimulation (dronabinol, a synthetic THC, is licensed as an appetite stimulant in patients with AIDS in the USA)
- Plants grown for fibre to produce paper, textiles and rope*
- Hempseed oil*

Potential medical uses
Limited evidence suggests cannabis resin (or extracts of it) could be used to treat the following:
- Glaucoma (cannabis has been prescribed for this purpose in the USA [32])
- Pain (there is increasing evidence for a role in this arena [33, 34])
- Multiple sclerosis (despite the poor quality of published research, which suggests a limited role for cannabis in alleviating MS symptoms, many sufferers claim that the resin can provide great relief [35])
- Epilepsy (cannabinol especially could be of some benefit [36, 37])
- Anxiety (cannabis is known to have anxiolytic actions [38])
- Infection (especially active against Gram-positive bacteria [39])

Historical uses
The following are defunct indications for use, which are no longer considered appropriate:
- Hysteria, depression, 'insanity', dementia
- Jaundice
- Venereal diseases
- Menorrhagia, dysmenorrhoea, difficult labour
- Gut spasm, flatulence, dysentry, cholera
- Tetanus, chorea, Parkinson's disease
- Cough
- Opioid withdrawal
- Aphrodisiac
- General anaesthetic
- Anthelminthic

*Varieties with a poor ability to produce resin are cultivated for these purposes.

population surveyed had used this drug [1]. In 1996, an investigation of the drug using habits of 7722 schoolchildren aged 15 to 16 years from around the UK revealed that 38.0 per cent of girls and 43.6 per cent of boys had taken cannabis at least once [2]. In the same year, an analysis of results from a study of 3075 second-year university students in the UK found that 55 per cent of women and 60 per cent of men had used cannabis at least once [3]. Nearly 20 per cent were regular users (at least once a week). The National Household Survey in the USA in both 1985 and 1992 showed that about 33 per cent of Americans had used cannabis at least once [4].

In general, the desired effects start within a few minutes of smoking and within one to three hours if ingested (depending on whether food is consumed at the same time). The duration of intoxication is determined by the dose and route. A small dose smoked may give effects lasting for only an hour whereas larger doses may last up to four hours. After oral administration the effects are more persistent and can last eight hours. As with most other drugs of abuse, the experience is largely determined by the surroundings and the mood, character and expectations of the user.

Cannabis commonly evokes elation and merriment in the initial stages, followed by relaxation, disinhibition and sociability. However, many first-time users report little or no effect. This may be due to inadequate dosage but there is also a high placebo response to cannabis. Regular users claim that one must know what to expect. Cannabis may produce heightened sensory awareness, enhanced imagination and time distortions. Only at high dosage will profound illusions or hallucinations appear – these are reported rarely.

ADMINISTRATION

The various forms of cannabis have different names. These are sometimes used interchangeably causing confusion over precise meaning, but the following details may be helpful:

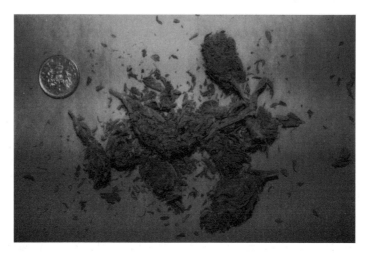

Figure 4.2 Dried *Cannabis* herb.

Marijuana

This term usually denotes the dried and crushed flower heads and small leaves of the cannabis plant (Figure 4.2). 'Marijuana' is actually the Hispanic spelling of the word and in American literature it is often written 'Marihuana'. The derivation is obscure. The term is more popular in the USA and is largely synonymous with slang terms such as grass, dope, weed, pot, hemp, bhang and ganja. Marijuana is sometimes used to describe the cannabis plant itself; the alternative is 'hash plant'. Cannabis herb prepared for use in this way contains about 0.5 to 2.5 per cent THC.

Hashish

The name hashish typically refers to the cannabis resin alone after removal from the plant; it is also known as hash (Figure 4.3). The term is derived from the Arabic *hashish al kief* (dried herb of pleasure). The colour and texture of the resin varies according to the geographical source and purity – it can be soft and putty-like, friable or hard, and red, yellow, brown or black in colour. It is typically brown with a toffee-like texture when pure. Hashish generally contains 2 to 8 per cent THC. Sinsemilla is the strongest variety of hashish, being derived from unfertilised female plants and containing up to 10 per cent THC.

Hash oil

Hash oil is a concentrated resin extract and the most potent form of cannabis used. The greenish-black viscous liquid can comprise 60 per cent or more THC.

In the UK, cannabis is nearly always smoked. Marijuana herb can be rolled into pure cigarettes or mixed with tobacco. These are called 'spliffs', 'joints' or 'reefers'. Hashish or hash oil is usually mixed with tobacco first because the amount needed to produce intoxication is quite small. The tobacco acts as a bulking agent and helps the cannabis to burn. Cannabis can also be smoked in a pipe. 'Hot knifing' is a method of burning the pure resin. A hot knife is passed through a block of resin so that some of its sticks and burns. The knife is then held under the nose so that the fumes can be inhaled.

Cannabis is also active when eaten or prepared as an infusion to drink. It has been a tradition for centuries in India, the Middle East and North Africa to take cannabis orally. The cannabis drink or sweetmeat must be flavoured to disguise the unpleasant taste of the crude resin.

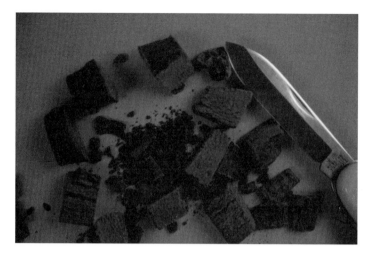

Figure 4.3 Cannabis resin.

Oral administration has not been popular elsewhere because psychoactive effects are slow to begin, unpredictable, can be blunted and are often of long duration.

PHARMACOKINETICS AND PHARMACOLOGY

THC is very lipophilic and after entering the lungs it dissolves quickly in pulmonary surfactant enabling rapid passage into the bloodstream. The high lipophilicity also facilitates quick penetration of the central nervous system (CNS) but the proportion of a dose which crosses the blood-brain barrier is low due to the high proportion of THC (97 per cent) which is bound to plasma proteins. THC distributes quickly into the adipose tissues of the body from which it is slowly released over time.

Oral doses are subject to extensive first-pass metabolism and rapid partition into body fat shortly after absorption, so despite almost complete absorption, only 10 to 20 per cent reaches the systemic circulation.

The initial (or alpha) half-life is about four hours and is a reflection of the rapid distribution of THC into adipose tissue. This is followed by a terminal (or beta) half-life of 25 to 36 hours as the drug is gradually released from body fat and metabolised. It may take several weeks for a single dose to be completely eliminated from the body. The main metabolite is 11-hydroxy-THC, which is formed in the liver and is also psychoactive. This is converted to 8,11-dehydroxy-THC before elimination. The majority of this metabolite is excreted in the bile, but there is some enterohepatic recycling. A small proportion (probably about one-fifth) is excreted in urine.

The mode of action of cannabis is not clear. There are a large number of cannabinoids and there may consequently be a range of different receptor types within the body. Two apparent receptor subtypes for THC have been located, one in the CNS and testes ('CB1') and one in the periphery ('CB2') [5]. An endogenous ligand for the CNS receptor has already been identified – anandamide [5]. This seems to have a role in central control of muscle movement, pain and anxiety regulation in animals. It also inhibits the secretion of follicle stimulating hormone and prolactin, as does THC.

ADVERSE EFFECTS

The adverse effects are summarised in Table 4.2. The precise effects of cannabis upon mental state vary considerably between individuals but are determined by the dose taken, the route of administration, the expectations of the user, the environment at the time of use, the concomitant use of other drugs, the user's emotional state and whether the individual is suffering from any psychiatric illness.

Cannabis intoxication can give rise to impaired judgement and incoordination, anxiety, dysphoria and confusion. Panic reactions and sedation can also occur. First-time users, in particular, may be especially prone to adverse mental effects, perhaps due to a lack of experience in dealing with the psychotropic effects of the drug. All of these effects on the CNS could increase the chance of accidents or risk-taking behaviour. Cannabis is also able to impair driving ability.

Paranoia and acute psychoses are well-known reactions [6–9]. The likelihood of all adverse mental effects increases as the dose increases. As with many other drugs of abuse it is very difficult to determine whether cases of psychiatric illness attributed to cannabis are true *de novo* drug-induced effects or whether cannabis simply unmasks a latent tendency to such illness. Whatever the mechanism, some individuals without a history of mental illness do experience short-lived, completely reversible, psychotic reactions lasting for a few days only. However, it is also known that cannabis can exacerbate symptoms of schizophrenia in those with pre-existing illness. 'Flashbacks' have been reported, but are much less common and more mild than those observed after using LSD.

Impairment of short-term memory occurs while intoxicated, as occurs with other inebriants such as alcohol. However, this effect may persist for several weeks beyond the period of acute intoxication

[1, 10, 11] although the duration of the effect and the extent of reversibility is unclear. The mechanism is also not understood.

Reddening of the whites of the eyes (especially after smoking) is a reaction which is frequently described. Another common side effect is coughing. Although acute inhalation of smoke containing cannabinoids may produce bronchodilation, the smoke is also irritant and can trigger bronchoconstriction in asthmatics. Abdominal pain, nausea and vomiting are sometimes reported.

Tachycardia is a common side effect; some users experience palpitations but arrhythmias are rare. Postural hypotension is a well-known cardiovascular side effect which is probably caused by dilatation of peripheral veins [12]. The transient cerebral ischaemia which results on assuming upright position can lead to dizziness and fainting. This may be at least partly due to impairment of the local regulation of cerebral blood flow [13]. Tachyphylaxis may develop to both orthostatic hypotension and tachycardia after regular administration. Facial flushing may occur in some users. Myocardial infarction (MI) has been reported as an adverse effect in a small number of case reports [14–17]. It is very difficult to know whether cannabis was responsible because of the numerous other variables which are known to predispose to MI. However, the patients involved were generally younger than the average MI sufferer.

LONG-TERM USE

Regular use of cannabis may encourage users to progress to other forms of drug abuse, although the likelihood of this occurring is more related to the lifestyle and personality of the individual than the effect of cannabis itself. Nonetheless the concept of cannabis as a 'gateway' to the use of other drugs of abuse is firmly established in the mind of the public. In a US telephone survey in 1995, 81 per cent of adolescents interviewed and 64 per cent of adults believed that a young person who used cannabis was more likely to progress to so-called harder drugs [18].

Chronic use is associated with an increase in airways resistance, an effect caused by an action on large airways [19]. This effect is not seen following tobacco smoking. The difference may be due to the way in which the two products are smoked. Cannabis smokers tend to take longer 'draws' and to inhale more deeply. It is also common practice to hold the breath for a few seconds after inhaling [20]. These actions may allow greater numbers of particles to reach the lower airways. The cannabis 'joint' is typically smoked to the very end of the butt, so that the smoke inhaled near the end contains more tar, carbon dioxide and particles and is also hotter [21]. A cannabis cigarette is home-made and so more loosely wrapped than a conventional tobacco cigarette; this may mean that fewer particles and tar are filtered out by the shaft of the cigarette itself. Cannabis cigarettes also do not contain filters. These features make the practice potentially more damaging to the airways. Cannabis cigarettes produce much more tar than tobacco varieties and, because of the way in which they are smoked, a greater proportion of this tar is retained in the lungs [20]. Consequently, the smoking of three or four cannabis 'joints' per day can produce the same degree of damage to the pulmonary epithelium as 20 or more tobacco cigarettes per day [22].

The smoking of cannabis can cause bronchitis or persistent sore throat but the link between cannabis smoking and lung cancer is not proven. This is a difficult subject to study because most users either smoke tobacco as well or use tobacco as a vehicle for smoking cannabis resin. The method of smoking cannabis described above may give any carcinogenic component a greater opportunity to operate on lung tissue because of the increased tissue contact time. The consensus of opinion is that because the risk of tobacco causing lung cancer is dose-related – and qualitatively the tar produced by a cannabis 'joint' is at least as toxic as that from a conventional cigarette – there must be at least some risk of lung cancer from smoking cannabis even if it is only due to the tobacco carrier. The risk is significantly reduced by the fact that most cannabis users are unlikely to smoke more than one 'joint' per day whereas most tobacco smokers consume at least 20 cigarettes over the same time period.

In one study, men who regularly used cannabis developed decreased testosterone levels and in some this was accompanied by a reduced sperm count [23]. However, most other studies have failed to confirm this effect on testosterone for reasons which are unclear [24]. In the 1st century AD, the Roman author Pliny wrote that cannabis could 'dry the seed of procreation'. Chronic use has even been claimed to cause gynaecomastia but few cases of this effect have been described [25]. Cannabis may cause impotence [24]. In female animals, cannabis inhibits ovulation and although this effect has been demonstrated in women it is unclear to what extent other confounding variables may have contributed to the observation [24]. Cannabis can reduce libido in both women and men [24].

The chronic effects of cannabinoids on the CNS are not clearly understood. Campbell et al. studied ten male subjects (average age 22) with significant cerebral atrophy, all of whom were chronic heavy cannabis users [26]. Subsequent studies using greater sophistication of technique (computerised tomography) have not confirmed these findings [27, 28] and cannabis is not now thought to cause cerebral damage.

Table 4.2   Adverse effects of cannabis

Acute effects
- Anxiety, confusion, drowsiness, panic reactions, psychosis, hallucinations, drowsiness, psychomotor impairment
- Red eyes
- Memory loss
- Tachycardia, palpitations, postural hypotension, flushing
- Coughing, sore throat, bronchospasm in asthmatic people
- Abdominal pain, nausea, vomiting

Effects from long-term use
- Bronchitis, ?lung cancer
- Oligospermia, gynaecomastia, decreased libido (both sexes)
- Insomnia, depression, anxiety, social withdrawal, decreased mental performance, reduced drive, 'flashbacks'
- Withdrawal symptoms on cessation

However, chronic use may be associated with insomnia, depression, dementia and anxiety [29]. Heavy daily abuse of most drugs tends to encourage social isolation and poor personal performance; the same is probably true of cannabis. An 'amotivational syndrome' has been described in certain chronic heavy users who seem unable to work towards desirable medium- or long-term objectives. They have a short attention span and can become introverted, apathetic and lacking in drive [29, 30]. Most researchers do not now believe that a distinct syndrome exists, as such, but some chronic users do become rather introspective. The French poet Charles Baudelaire, who took cannabis himself, wrote a discourse entitled 'The Poem of Hashish' in 1846. In it, he makes the following observation:

> But can the drug be said to be truly devoid of side effects when it renders the individual useless to Society and Society unnecessary to the individual?

People who abuse cannabis regularly at high dose may experience withdrawal symptoms on cessation [25]. These include anxiety, irritability, deranged appetite, poor sleep, restlessness, hot flushes and rhinorrhoea. Similar reactions have been described after discontinuation of high-dose therapeutic cannabinoids such as oral dronabinol 210 mg per day for 12 to 16 days [31]. In cannabis smokers the effect is seen infrequently and it is generally considered to be a drug with a very low dependence potential. Tolerance to the psychoactive effects or physical dependence are unlikely to occur unless there is sustained heavy exposure every day for a long time. Varying degrees of 'psychological' dependence are more common and characterised by a strong desire for continued cannabis use but not accompanied by a withdrawal syndrome. The following criteria for diagnosis of cannabis dependence have been proposed [29]:

(a) preoccupation with obtaining supplies of cannabis;
(b) compulsion to take cannabis, despite adverse consequences;
(c) relapse to regular use of cannabis following attempted abstinence.

The majority of cannabis users seem to be able to stop taking the preparation easily without complications. In fact, the majority are occasional users rather than daily habituées.

REFERENCES

1. Deahl, M. (1991) Cannabis and memory loss (editorial). *Br. J. Addiction*, **86**: 249–252.
2. Miller, P.McC. and Plant, M. (1996) Drinking, smoking and illicit drug use among 15 and 16 year olds in the United Kingdom. *Br. Med. J.* **313**: 394–397.
3. Webb, E., Ashton, C.H., Kelly, P. and Kamali, F. (1996) Alcohol and drug use in UK university students. *Lancet*, **348**: 922–925.
4. Anon (1995) Marijuana Update, *NIDA Capsule (CAP12)*. National Institute on Drug Abuse, USA, p.1.
5. Musty, R.E., Reggio, P. and Consroe, P. (1995) A review of recent advances in cannabinoid research and the 1994 international symposium on cannabis and the cannabinoids. *Life Sci.* **56**: 1933–1940.
6. Rottanburg, D., Ben-Arie, O., Robins, A.H., Teggin, A. and Elk, R. (1982) Cannabis-associated psychosis with hypomanic features. *Lancet*, **ii**: 1364–1366.
7. Andreasson, S., Allebeck, P., Engstrom, A. and Rydberg, U. (1987) Cannabis and schizophrenia – a longitudinal study of Swedish conscripts. *Lancet*, **ii**: 1483–1485.
8. Wylie, A.S., Scott, R.T.A. and Burnett, S.J. (1995) Psychosis due to 'skunk' (letter). *Br. Med. J.* **311**: 125.
9. McBride, A.J. and Thomas, H. (1995) Psychosis is also common in users of 'normal' cannabis (letter). *Br. Med. J.* **311**: 875.
10. Schwartz, R.H., Gruenewald, P.J., Klitzner, M. and Fedio, P. (1989) Short-term memory impairment in cannabis-dependent adolescents. *Am. J. Dis. Child.* **143**: 1214–1219.
11. Pope, H.G. and Yurgelun-Todd, D. (1996) The residual cognitive effects of heavy marijuana use in college students. *J. Am. Med. Assoc.* **275**: 521–527.

12. Merritt, J.C. (1982) Orthostatic hypotension after delta-9-tetrahydro-cannabinol marihuana inhalation. *Ophthal. Res.* **14**: 124–128.

13. Mathew, R.J., Wilson, W.H., Humphreys, D., Lowe, J.V. and Wiethe, K.E. (1992) Middle cerebral artery velocity during upright posture after marijuana smoking. *Acta Psychiatr. Scand.* **86**: 173–178.

14. Collins, J.S.A., Higginson, J.D.S., Boyle, D.M.C. and Webb, S.W. (1985) Myocardial infarction during marijuana smoking in a young female. *Eur. Heart J.* **6**: 637–638.

15. Macinnes, D.C. and Miller, K.M. (1984) Fatal coronary artery thrombosis associated with cannabis smoking. *J. R. Coll. Gen. Prac.* **34**: 575–576.

16. Coutselinis, A. and Michalodimitrakis, M. (1981) Myocardial infarction and marijuana. *Clin. Toxicol.* **18**: 389–390.

17. Pearl, W. and Choi, Y.S. (1992) Marijuana as a cause of myocardial infarction (letter). *Int. J. Cardiol.* **34**: 353.

18. News (1995) Teens cite illicit drugs as major worry, see marijuana as gateway. *Am. J. Health. Syst. Pharm.* **52**: 2170, 2174.

19. Tashkin, D.P., Coulson, A.H., Clark, V.A. *et al.* (1987) Respiratory symptoms and lung function in habitual heavy smokers of marijuana alone, smokers of marijuana and tobacco, smokers of tobacco alone, and nonsmokers. *Am. Rev. Resp. Dis.* **135**: 209–216.

20. Wu, T-Z., Tashkin, D.P., Djahed, B. and Rose, J.E. (1988) Pulmonary hazards of smoking marijuana compared with tobacco. *N. Engl. J. Med.* **318**: 347–351.

21. Tashkin, D.P., Gliederer, F., Rose, J. *et al.* (1991) Tar, CO, and delta-9-THC delivery from the 1st and 2nd halves of a marijuana cigarette. *Pharmacol. Biochem. Behav.* **40**: 657–661.

22. Gong, H., Fligiel, S., Tashkin, D.P. and Barbers, R.G. (1987) Tracheobronchial changes in habitual, heavy smokers of marijuana with and without tobacco. *Am. Rev. Resp. Dis.* **136**: 142–149.

23. Kolodny, R.C., Masters, W.H., Kolodner, R. and Toro, G. (1974) Depression of plasma testosterone levels after chronic intensive marihuana use. *N. Engl. J. Med.* **290**: 872–874.

24. Abel, E.L. (1981) Marihuana and sex: a critical survey. *Drug Alcohol Depend.* **8**: 1–22.

25. Harmon, J. and Aliapoulios, M.A. (1972) Gynecomastia in marihuana users (letter). *N. Engl. J. Med.* **287**: 936.

26. Campbell, A.M.G., Evans, M., Thomson, J.L.G. and Williams, M.J. (1971) Cerebral atrophy in young cannabis smokers. *Lancet,* **ii**: 1219–1225.

27. Co, B., Goodwin, D.W., Gado, M., Mikhael, M. and Hill, S.Y. (1977) Absence of cerebral atrophy in chronic cannabis users by computerized transaxial tomography. *J. Am. Med. Assoc.* **237**: 1229–1230.

28. Kuehnle, J., Mendelson, J.H., Davis, K.R. and New, P.F.J. (1977) Computed tomographic examination of heavy marihuana smokers.

J. Am. Med. Assoc. **237**: 1231–1232.

29. Miller, N.S. and Gold, M.S. (1989) The diagnosis of marijuana (cannabis) dependence. *J Subst. Abuse Treat.* **6**: 183–192.

30. Weller, R.A. (1985) Marijuana: effects and motivation. *Med. Aspects Human Sexuality*, **19**: 92–105.

31. Anon. (1995) *Marinol (dronabinol) Product Information.* Physicians' Desk Reference. Medical Economics, Montvale, NJ, pp. 2129–2131.

32. Hepler, R.S., Frank, I.M. and Petrus, R. (1976) Ocular effects of marihuana smoking, in *The Pharmacology of Marihuana*, (eds M.C. Braude and S. Szara), Raven Press, New York, pp.815–819.

33. Noyes, R., Brunk, F., Avery, D.H. and Canter, A. (1975) The analgesic properties of delta-9-tetrahydrocannabinol and codeine. *Clin. Pharmacol. Ther.* **18**: 84–89.

34. Noyes, R., Brunk, F., Baram. D.A. and Canter, A. (1976) Analgesic effects of delta-9-tetrahydrocannabinol. *The Pharmacology of Marihuana*, (eds M.C. Braude and S. Szara), Raven Press, New York, pp. 833–836.

35. Wills, S. (1995) The use of cannabis in multiple sclerosis. *Pharm. J.* **255**: 237–238.

36. Carlini, E.A. and Cunha, J.M. (1981) Hypnotic and antiepileptic effects of cannabidiol. *J. Clin. Pharmacol.* **21(suppl)**: 417S–427S.

37. Consroe, P.F., Wood, G.C. and Buchsbaum, H. (1975) Anticonvulsant nature of marihuana smoking. *J. Am. Med. Assoc.* **234**: 306–307.

38. Nakano, S., Gillespie, H.K. and Hollister, L.E. (1978) A model for evaluation of anti-anxiety drugs with the use of experimentally induced stress: Comparison of nabilone and diazepam. *Clin. Pharmacol. Ther.* **23**: 54–62.

39. Radosevic, A., Kupinic, M. and Grilic, L. (1962) Antibiotic activity of various types of cannabis resin. *Nature*, **195**: 1007–1009.

5

Cocaine

Save for the occasional use of Cocaine he had no vices, and he only turned to the drug as a protest against the monotony of existence . . .
Dr Watson describing Sherlock Holmes in
'The Adventure of the Yellow Face',
Sir Arthur Conan Doyle, 1893.

HISTORY

Cocaine occurs naturally in the leaves of the coca plant, *Erythroxylum coca*, and certain related species which originate from South America, especially Peru, Bolivia and Colombia. The Incas considered the plant a divine gift and reserved its use for the higher echelons of society. Conversely, all levels of society amongst the Andean Indians have used the leaves as a masticatory for thousands of years. The leaves are combined with slaked lime or plant ash to produce an alkaline medium which enables the cocaine base to form a solution in saliva and thus enter the circulation. Chewing the leaves helps the Indians tolerate hunger, exposure and fatigue at high altitudes where the working environment can be hostile. Cocaine provides a stimulus to manual labour, therefore, as well as inducing feelings of pleasure. The leaves contain about 1 per cent cocaine.

In about 1860, cocaine was isolated and identified as the active constituent of the coca plant. It was subsequently employed medicinally as a local anaesthetic. Karl Köller was probably the first to use it in humans, when he performed eye surgery in 1884.

When recreational use of cocaine developed outside South America, the form developed was a water-soluble extract: crystalline cocaine hydrochloride. This is still probably the form of drug most widely used;

it is often mixed with a diluent powder on the street and in the UK is usually known as coke, snow or blow.

Until relatively recently, cocaine was viewed in the UK as an expensive drug, used more by the wealthier sections of the population. However, the number of abusers at all levels of society has increased. This is probably because cocaine has a reputation as a 'clean' drug and the street price has decreased considerably. Other factors influencing the greater demand for the drug may include the increased availability of very pure forms of cocaine such as 'crack' and the fact that various forms of the drug can produce rapid-onset, short-lived but intense effects without the need for injection.

'Crack' is a highly pure form of the free base of cocaine (i.e. it is not a salt of cocaine like cocaine hydrochloride). The name is thought to originate from the cracking noises that lumps of free base make when heated up. This noise is probably caused by impurities in the cocaine remaining from the extraction process (e.g. sodium bicarbonate, sodium chloride). 'Crack' began to be available on a large scale in the USA in the mid-1980s (Figure 5.1).

EFFECTS SOUGHT

When cocaine is injected or 'crack' is smoked, users hope to experience a 'rush' of exhilaration as the drug reaches the brain. This is afforded by rapid access to the circulation. It is not a feature of nasal insufflation of the hydrochloride salt because absorption across the

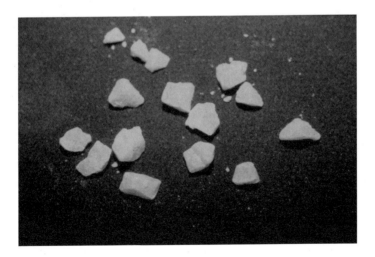

Figure 5.1 'Crack' cocaine.

nasal mucous membranes is slow (it is probably further retarded by the vasoconstrictor actions of cocaine which restrict blood flow to the site).

The desired effects of cocaine are heralded by a series of adrenaline-like reactions due to stimulation of the sympathetic nervous system and release of adrenaline. Generally the mental effects produced by cocaine are feelings of euphoria, alertness, excitement and rapid flow of thought. This may manifest as hyperactivity, increased confidence, talkativeness and sometimes emotional lability. When intoxicated, abusers may feel indifferent to matters which normally cause them great concern.

Cocaine is a stimulant; it helps to combat fatigue and subjectively there may be feelings of increased capacity to do work, great physical strength and mental supremacy.

ADMINISTRATION

The usual method of use for cocaine hydrochloride is to arrange the powder in a line on a flat surface and inhale it nasally via a small tube (e.g. a drinking straw or rolled paper). This method of nasal insufflation is termed 'snorting'. Cocaine hydrochloride powder is illustrated in Figure 5.2.

The hydrochloride salt has a high melting point (197°C) and it is not very stable when heated to high temperature. It is therefore costly and wasteful to smoke because large amounts need to be used. The free base form of cocaine has greater thermal stability and a lower melting point (98°C), making it a more suitable preparation to smoke. The

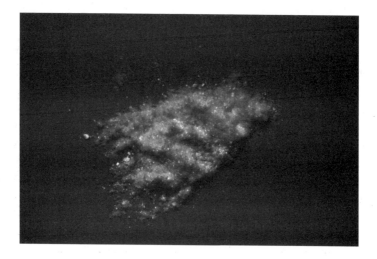

Figure 5.2 Cocaine hydrochloride powder.

method of production involves treating cocaine hydrochloride with alkali, followed by the heating of the precipitate in a glass pipe. The alkaloid base vapour is then inhaled. This technique is called 'freebasing'.

'Crack' cocaine is ready-made free base cocaine which has been prepared on a large scale and sold on the street. 'Crack' may be smoked in a pipe, heated on foil and the vapour inhaled, or smoked with tobacco in a cigarette.

Injection of cocaine is a less popular method of abuse than smoking or insufflation. The hydrochloride is generally used because it is much more water-soluble than 'crack'. However, in one study over 20 per cent of 'crack' users were found to be attempting injection of the free base [1]. The time to onset of action and peak effects are similar to those seen with 'crack' smoking. A 'speedball' is a mixed injection of heroin and cocaine favoured by some abusers.

Cocaine is active when taken orally but is not commonly taken by this route because the onset of action is too slow and the effects are much less intense.

When an abuser 'freebases', smokes 'crack' or injects cocaine hydrochloride, the psychoactive effects begin within seconds but peak after a few minutes. To maintain the desired euphoria the process must be repeated frequently. Repeated use of drug in this way is described as a 'run' or a 'binge'. It may continue until the individual is exhausted or until the supply of drug runs out. The peak effects from nasal insufflation or oral administration take longer to develop: 15 to 30 minutes for nasal insufflation, up to an hour when taken orally. Hence abuse via these routes is less likely to be associated with a 'run'. After a 'run' or a single dose, an individual may 'crash', i.e. experience post-cocaine dysphoria.

PHARMACOKINETICS AND PHARMACOLOGY

The half-life of cocaine varies from 45 to 90 minutes [2, 3]. The average is probably about 60 minutes. There may be a moderate increase in half-life as the dose increases [3]. The psychotropic effects of the drug last for varying lengths of time depending on the method of administration. These differences are summarised in Table 5.1.

The majority of a cocaine dose (about 90 per cent) is metabolised by hydrolysis. Plasma and liver pseudocholinesterases convert cocaine to metabolites which may have some action on the sympathetic nervous system but which are not thought to be psychoactive. The three major metabolites are ecgonine methyl ester, benzoylecgonine and ecgonine [4]. These are excreted in urine. The remaining proportion which is not

Table 5.1 Time course of psychoactive effects of cocaine

Form of cocaine	Administration method	Time to peak effects	Duration of effects
Hydrochloride	Intravenous	< 5 min	30–45 min
Hydrochloride	'Snorted'	10–15 min	60–90 min
'Crack'	Smoked	< 15 s	15–20 min

hydrolysed is metabolised in the liver by N-demethylation. The ultimate product of this metabolic pathway, norcocaine nitroxide, has been proposed as the cause of cocaine-induced hepatotoxicity [5] (but see below).

Cocaine inhibits reuptake of dopamine, noradrenaline and serotonin in central and peripheral nerve synapses and so effectively prolongs and augments their effects. It seems particularly to increase the concentration of neurotransmitters in dopaminergic areas of the brain. The inhibition of dopamine reuptake is believed to cause euphoria and this is the main reason why users continue to take the drug. Mice which have been genetically manipulated so that they lack a central dopamine reuptake mechanism at synapses do not respond to cocaine at all [6]. Cocaine may also increase the release of noradrenaline into sympathetic nervous system synapses and stimulate the release of adrenaline from the adrenals.

In the laboratory setting many experienced abusers, given unidentified drugs to inject, cannot distinguish between the effects of cocaine and those of amphetamine. This is not surprising as they produce similar net effects at the synapse level but by different mechanisms. Both drugs increase the activity of similar central nervous system (CNS) neurotransmitters, have stimulant properties and enhance the peripheral sympathetic nervous system. Their similarity is further supported by study of side effect profiles which are remarkably alike.

ADVERSE EFFECTS

As with many drugs of abuse, the most serious side effects are often a consequence of acute overdosage or chronic use of high doses. Potential acute adverse reactions, occurring within a few hours of taking cocaine, are summarised in Table 5.2. There is no specific treatment for cocaine intoxication *per se*.

The cardiac toxicity of cocaine has been studied in some detail because many deaths have been attributed to this adverse effect. The effects upon the heart in any one person are unpredictable but cocaine

Table 5.2   Acute adverse reactions to cocaine

- Adrenaline-like effects such as tachycardia, mydriasis, sweating, tremor, flushing, reduced appetite, headaches
- Nausea and vomiting
- Chest pain, black sputum, wheeziness, shortness of breath, respiratory arrest
- Hypertension, palpitations, tachyarrhythmias, myocarditis, cardiomyopathy, cardiac arrest, sudden death
- Stroke, convulsions
- Rhabdomyolysis [43], with or without hyperpyrexia, and sequelae
- Anxiety, paranoia, hallucinations (visual, auditory, tactile) after large doses. Acute psychotic reactions, panic reactions, violence [44]
- Cocaine may induce heightened sexual interest; this may result in acquisition of sexually transmitted diseases or unwanted pregnancies
- Intoxication may facilitate accidents or participation in risk-taking behaviour [45]
- After a 'run' there is frequently a 'crash', characterised by dysphoria, depression, irritability and craving for the drug; this is often followed by fatigue and sleep

has been reported to cause a variety of cardiac adverse effects [7–11] (see Table 5.2), of which myocardial infarction (MI) is the most serious. MI has been documented in numerous case reports and the likelihood of infarction does not seem to be related to duration of use, frequency of use or method of administration.

In patients with pre-existing ischaemic heart disease, cocaine can have an apparently sympathomimetic effect on the heart, increasing myocardial oxygen demands to the extent that angina pains occur and sometimes myocardial infarction. However, the majority of patients who have suffered a heart attack as a result of taking cocaine do not have pre-existing symptomatic heart disease and a thrombus is often absent at post-mortem. Research has shown that cocaine can cause coronary vasospasm [12–16]. The exact mechanism of this is uncertain, but it could be a direct vasoconstriction caused by cocaine itself or the catecholamines that it can release. Cocaine abuse can cause endothelial damage, and vasospasm could consequently be at least partly due to a reduction in the synthesis of endothelium-derived vasodilators such as nitric oxide or prostacyclin. However, it seems unlikely that coronary vasospasm alone would be sufficient to trigger a fatal infarction. The effect may be augmented by formation of a thrombus which lyses before post-mortem (platelet aggregation being triggered by the aforementioned damage to the endothelium) and catecholamine-induced increase in myocardial oxygen requirement.

In one study, coronary vasospasm closely mirrored the time course of cocaine plasma levels. But spasm also occurred when there was a later peak in cocaine metabolites, so these may also be important in the aetiology of cocaine cardiotoxicity [15].

Arrhythmias produced by cocaine may simply be secondary to the adrenergic effects of the drug. However, arrhythmias could arise as a result of the adverse cardiac effects of cocaine (MI, myocarditis or the reperfusion after coronary artery spasm). Cocaine as a local anaesthetic also has direct membrane stabilising effects on the myocardium itself and can be demonstrated to prolong the QT interval on an electrocardiogram (ECG).

Chest pain is quite a common complaint. A study of 217 chronic 'crack' smokers showed that 39 per cent suffered pains in the chest within an hour of smoking cocaine; 64 per cent reported a pain that was made worse by taking a deep breath [17]. The cause of the pain is unclear; there may be more than one kind of pain and therefore a variety of causes. The pain is generally short-lived. It can be due to cocaine-induced MI or cardiac ischaemia but when a series of 100 chest pain patients were given an ECG, only 8 per cent had a trace typical of an MI [18]. Researchers have suggested inflammation of pleural membranes as a cause because of the pain on inspiration [17]. Thoracic muscle rhabdomyolysis has also been suggested [18, 19] and this is consistent with the high creatinine kinase levels observed in such patients. Involvement of pectoral or intercostal muscles would explain why the pain can be more intense on inspiration. In those taking amphetamine derivatives similar pains have been attributed to spasm of the intercostal muscles [20]. It is not known how cocaine could be toxic to skeletal muscle. If it is capable of causing prolonged spasm this could give rise to rhabdomyolysis, although why thoracic muscles alone should be specifically involved is not understood.

Cocaine 'snorting' or smoking can exacerbate asthma. Rubin and Neugarten described six asthmatics who suffered severe or life-threatening bronchospasm after using cocaine [21]. Wheezing has been described in up to a third of free base smokers [22]. A US study of 217 chronic smokers of the free base revealed that 44 per cent of subjects had reported coughing up black sputum within 12 hours of use and that 6 per cent had coughed up blood [17]. Other pulmonary complications appear to be very rare but include pulmonary oedema, pneumomediastinum, pneumothorax and bronchiolitis [23].

Stroke is rare in patients under 45 years of age but the taking of cocaine is associated with an increased risk [24–26]. Haemorrhagic stroke is more likely than thrombotic or embolic types.

Convulsions are probably more common when high doses, or long 'runs' of cocaine are used. Fitting can occur with any mode of administration and seems to resolve without leaving a permanent propensity to seizures, whether treated with anticonvulsants or not [26-29].

LONG-TERM USE

Panic attacks are a common acute psychiatric problem. But chronic cocaine abuse may cause a range of psychiatric problems which may be acute or chronic. Anxiety, nervousness, depression, exhaustion, mania and paranoid psychosis have all been attributed to frequent cocaine use [26, 30, 31]. Persistent anhedonia or dysphoria can also develop. Subjects may find it difficult to concentrate, suffer from memory loss and become antisocial. The anorexic properties of the drug frequently give rise to weight loss.

Perforation of the nasal septum and rhinorrhoea commonly result from regular 'snorting' of cocaine. However, the effects on the rest of the respiratory tract are less clear. Chronic abusers often have a cough and may suffer from bouts of wheeziness or a hoarse voice. Measurements of lung function can reveal a deterioration in the gaseous exchange capacity of the alveoli but the implications of this for long-term health are not understood.

Dental erosions have been reported in those who draw snorted cocaine through the nose and then into the mouth, thus partly relying on buccal absorption. This is more likely to occur in those with a perforated nasal septum. The high salivary pH caused by cocaine is thought to be responsible for the resulting damage to teeth [32].

Despite cocaine being a dose-dependent hepatotoxin in mice [33], it is unclear whether the drug has a similar effect in humans. A review by Farrell highlighted that, in all reported cases of alleged cocaine-induced liver damage, more obvious well-established causes of liver failure were either present or had not been excluded [34]. Farrell suggested that hepatic ischaemia caused by shock and hypotension were more likely mechanisms by which cocaine could derange liver function than a direct hepatotoxic action of cocaine or its metabolite norcocaine nitroxide.

Limited studies suggest that cocaine may accelerate the process of atheroma formation [8] and cases of thrombocytopenia occurring up to three weeks after use have also been reported [35].

Dependence

Cocaine can produce both physical and psychological dependence but the dependence potential of cocaine may vary according to the method of administration. 'Snorting' cocaine hydrochloride has a lower dependence potential than smoking the free base ('crack') or injecting the hydrochloride. This is probably because these latter two methods cause such an intense and short-lived exhilaration. In animal studies, cocaine possesses very potent 'reinforcing properties', i.e. animals will more quickly adopt a certain pattern of behaviour if cocaine is offered as a reward. In humans this is manifested as a 'craving' for the drug. The individual has a strong desire to experience again the euphoric effects of the drug (positive reinforcement) and may also be driven by the desire to reverse the dysphoric aftermath (negative reinforcement). Positive reinforcement is probably the dominant drive to continued use. 'Crack' cocaine has been associated with a particularly strong craving; heavy users may go without food or sleep for long periods in order to continue to use the drug.

Craving may persist for weeks after cessation of chronic administration and is the most prominent feature of withdrawal. Sometimes other symptoms of withdrawal are seen including irritability, depression, anxiety, insomnia and dysphoria. Craving encourages the subject to continue the abuse but, unlike opioid withdrawal, there seem to be no physiological signs necessitating a gradual reduction in the dose of the drug.

Treatment

Pharmacologically, a variety of drugs have been used in an attempt to reduce cocaine use, decrease craving and alleviate dependence or symptoms of withdrawal. Research has concentrated mainly on two approaches. In the first, antidepressants have been used because cocaine abstinence produces symptoms similar to depression. The second popular approach has been to employ drugs which interact with dopamine because this neurotransmitter is known to have a key role in the positive reinforcement produced by cocaine. Other pharmacological approaches have involved drugs which affect neurotransmitters which may be involved in the neurochemical effects of cocaine (e.g. serotonin, opioids) and symptomatic treatment of underlying mental illness. Non-pharmacological approaches are important and include counselling, behavioural therapy and psychotherapy. These are beyond the scope of this book, but are reviewed elsewhere [36, 37].

Tricyclic antidepressants, particularly desipramine, seem to facilitate an initial abstinence from cocaine and this initial success may be independent of whether the individual suffers from depression or not [38, 39]. However, the continued success of treatment may be related to the existence of underlying depression. It has been suggested that tricyclics only be used for six to ten weeks in those without depression because otherwise side effects such as jitteriness and stimulation may act as cues for cocaine craving [39]. In those who do suffer from depression, it may be beneficial to continue tricyclics in order to prevent recurrence of depression which could otherwise encourage a desire for the mood-elevating effects of cocaine. Identifying depression in drug abusers can be difficult, not least because cocaine itself can be a cause of depression. Desipramine is more successful in cocaine abusers than in chronic cocaine dependents [40].

Patients with schizophrenia who abuse cocaine [39] may need bigger doses of existing treatment or a complete reappraisal of neuroleptic therapy if cocaine has exacerbated psychosis. Alternatively, such patients may require specific treatment for neuroleptic adverse reactions if cocaine is being taken to counteract these effects. This may necessitate reduced doses of existing treatment, a change in neuroleptic or an additional drug (e.g. an antimuscarinic). If cocaine is being taken simply as a mood enhancer, an antidepressant may help (as above).

Studies have suggested that buprenorphine may reduce cocaine use [40, 41]. This effect could be because central opioid pathways may help mediate cocaine dependence but also because many cocaine abusers use, or are dependent upon, opioids at the same time. Bromocriptine may decrease craving and dysphoria in some individuals [40, 41] but side-effects are troublesome. Carbamazepine and fluoxetine have been studied but are probably ineffective.

Social and environmental 'cues' are important in triggering craving for cocaine; at the physiological level dopamine may be the neurotransmitter involved in this effect. A recent small study of 20 patients suggested that a dopamine antagonist such as haloperidol 4 mg daily could reduce craving [42]. This is important because cue-elicited craving is one of the main reasons for recidivism in cocaine dependents seeking abstinence.

Recent work in animals has suggested that stimulation of post-synaptic dopamine D1 receptors can prevent or alleviate craving for cocaine whereas stimulation of D2 receptors may actually increase craving [6]. A highly specific D1 agonist that has no activity at other dopamine receptors could therefore be very helpful therapeutically. In 1995, a team of researchers showed that it was possible to vaccinate against the action of cocaine in rats such that CNS concentrations and response to the drug were markedly reduced [6].

For cocaine abusers and dependents there are no universally applicable pharmacological interventions which will aid abstinence, prevent craving or treat withdrawal. Most users of cocaine seeking abstinence simply stop taking the drug abruptly, with or without counselling or other non-pharmacological support. There is no necessity to medicate the immediate withdrawal period, but drugs such as desipramine may make it easier for some. Unless there is a treatable 'reason' for abuse (e.g. depression), there are no drugs to stop the chronic compulsion to take cocaine. Hence the chronic cocaine abuser must unfortunately rely largely on 'will power' to prevent recidivism.

REFERENCES

1. Pickering, H., Donoghoe, M., Green, A. and Foster, R. (1993) Crack injection. *Druglink*, **8**: 12.
2. Resnick, R.B., Kestenbaum, R.S. and Schwartz, L.K. (1977) Acute systemic effects of cocaine in man – a controlled study by intranasal and intravenous routes. *Science*, **195**: 696–698.
3. Jones, R.T. (1984) The pharmacology of cocaine. *NIDA Res. Monogr.* **50**: 27–34.
4. Stewart, D.J., Inaba, T., Lucassen, M. and Kalow, W. (1979) Cocaine and norcocaine hydrolysis by liver and serum esterases. *Clin. Pharmacol. Ther.* **25**: 464–468.
5. Kloss, M.W., Rosen, G.M. and Rauckman, E.J. (1984) Cocaine mediated hepatotoxicity. A critical review. *Biochem. Pharmacol.* **33**: 169–173.
6. Leshner, A.I. (1996) Molecular mechanisms of cocaine addiction. *N. Engl. J. Med.* **335**: 128–129.
7. Thadani, P. (ed) (1991) Cardiovascular toxicity of cocaine: underlying mechanisms. *NIDA Res. Monogr.* **108**.
8. Om, A. (1992) Cardiovascular complications of cocaine. *Am. J. Med. Sci.* **303**: 333–339.
9. Kloner, R.A., Hale, S., Alker, K. and Rezkalla, S. (1992) The effects of acute and chronic cocaine use on the heart. *Circulation*, **85**: 407–419.
10. VanDette, J.M. and Cornish, L.A. (1989) Medical complications of illicit cocaine use. *Clin. Pharmacol.* **8**: 401–411.
11. Om, A., Ellahham, S. and DiSciascio, G. (1993) Management of cocaine-induced cardiovascular complications. *Am. Heart. J.* **124**: 469–475.
12. Virmani, R. (1991) Cocaine-associated cardiovascular disease: clinical and pathological aspects. *NIDA Res. Monogr.* **108**: 220–229.
13. Isner, J.M. and Chokshi, S.K. (1991) Cocaine-induced myocardial infarction: clinical observations and pathogenetic considerations. *NIDA Res. Monogr.* **108**: 121–130.

14. Minor, R.L., Brook, D.S., Brown, D.B. and Winniford, M.D. (1991) Cocaine-induced myocardial infarction in patients with normal coronary arteries. *Ann. Intern. Med.* **115**: 797–806.

15. Brogan III, W.C., Lange, R.A., Glamann, D.B. and Hillis, L.D. (1992) Recurrent coronary vasoconstriction caused by intranasal cocaine: possible role for metabolites. *Ann. Intern. Med.* **116**: 556–561.

16. Lange, R.A., Cigarroa, R.G., Yancy Jr, C.W. *et al.* (1989) Cocaine-induced coronary artery vasoconstriction. *N. Engl. J. Med.* **321**: 1557–1562.

17. Khalsa, M.E., Tashkin, D.P. and Perrochet, B. (1992) Smoked cocaine: patterns of use and pulmonary consequences. *J. Psychoactive Drugs*, **24**: 265–272.

18. Gitter, M.J., Goldsmith, S.R., Dunbar, D.N. and Sharkey, S.W. (1991) Cocaine and chest pain: clinical features and outcome of patients hospitalized to rule out myocardial infarction. *Ann. Intern. Med.* **115**: 277–282.

19. Rubin, R.B. and Neugarten, J. (1989) Cocaine-induced rhabdomyolysis masquerading as myocardial ischaemia. *Am. J. Med.* **86**: 551–553.

20. Rittoo, D., Rittoo, D.B. and Rittoo, D. (1992) Misuse of ecstasy (letter). *Br. Med. J.* **305**: 309–310.

21. Rubin, R.B. and Neugarten, J. (1990) Cocaine-associated asthma (letter). *Am. J. Med.* **88**: 438–439.

22. Suhl, J. and Gorelick, D.A. (1988) Pulmonary function in male free base cocaine smokers (abstract). *Am. J. Resp. Dis.* **137**: 488.

23. Ettinger, N.A. and Albin, R.J. (1989) A review of the respiratory effects of smoking cocaine. *Am. J. Med.* **87**: 664–668.

24. Klonoff, D.C. (1989) Stroke associated with cocaine use. *Arch. Neurol.* **46**: 989–993.

25. Kaku, D.A. and Lowenstein, D.H. (1990) Emergence of recreational drug abuse as a major risk factor for stroke in young adults. *Ann. Intern. Med.* **113**: 821–827.

26. Miller, B.L., Mena, I., Giombetti, R., Villanueva-Meyer, J. and Djenderedjian, A.H. (1992) Neuropsychiatric effects of cocaine: SPECT measurements. *J. Addict. Dis.* **11**: 47–58.

27. Shallash, A.J., Shih, R.D., Hoffman, R.S., Holland III, R.W. and Marx, J.A. (1993) Grand mal seizures and cocaine use. *Ann. Emerg. Med.* **22**: 758.

28. Harden, C.L., Daras, M. and Tuchman, A.J. (1992) Cocaine causing convulsions in a large municipal hospital population. *J. Epilepsy*, **5**: 175–177.

29. Holland III, R.W., Marx, J.A., Earnest, M.P. and Rannoiger, S. (1992) Grand mal seizures temporally related to cocaine use: clinical and diagnostic features. *Ann. Emerg. Med.* **21**: 772–776.

30. Lacayo, A. (1995) Neurologic and psychiatric complications of cocaine abuse. *Neuropsychiatr. Neuropsychol. Behav. Neurol.* **8**: 53–60.

31. Brady, K.T., Lydiard, R.B., Malcolm, R. and Ballenger, J.C. (1991) Cocaine-induced psychosis. *J. Clin. Psychiatr.* **52**: 509–512.

32. Krutchkoff, D.J., Eisenberg, E., O'Brien, J.E. and Ponzillo, J.J. (1990) Cocaine-induced dental erosions (letter). *N. Engl. J. Med.* **322**: 408.

33. Evans, M.A. and Harbison, R.D. (1978) Cocaine-induced hepatotoxicity in mice. *Toxicol. Appl. Pharmacol.* **45**: 739–754.

34. Farrell, G.C. (1994) *Drug-induced Liver Disease*, Churchill Livingstone, London, pp. 236–239.

35. Leissinger, C.A. (1990) Severe thrombocytopenia associated with cocaine use. *Ann. Intern. Med.* **112**: 708–710.

36. Higgins, S.T., Budney, A.J. and Bickel, W.K. (1994) Applying behavioral concepts and principles to the treatment of cocaine dependence. *Drug Alcohol Depend.* **34**: 87–97.

37. Carroll, K.M. (1993) Psychotherapeutic treatment of cocaine abuse: models for its evaluation alone and in combination with pharmacotherapy. *NIDA Res. Monogr.* **135**: 116–132.

38. Gawin, F.H., Kleber, H.D., Byck, R. *et al.* (1989) Desipramine facilitation of initial cocaine abstinence. *Arch. Gen. Psychiatr.* **46**: 117–121.

39. Schottenfeld, R., Carroll, K. and Rounsaville, B. (1993) Comorbid psychiatric disorders and cocaine abuse. *NIDA Res. Monogr.* **135**: 31–47.

40. Mendelson, J.H. and Mello, N.K. (1996) Management of cocaine abuse and dependence. *N. Engl. J. Med.* **334**: 965–972.

41. Kleber, H.D., Tamminga, C.A., Schreur, B. *et al.* (1995) Pharmacotherapy, current and potential, for the treatment of cocaine dependence. *Clin. Neuropharmacol.* **18(suppl. 1)**: S96–S109.

42. Berger, S.P., Mickalian, J.D., Reid, M.S. *et al.* (1996) Haloperidol antagonism of cue-elicited cocaine craving. *Lancet*, **347**: 504–508.

43. Roth, D., Alarcon, F.J., Fernandez, J.A. *et al.* (1988) Acute rhabdomyolysis associated with cocaine intoxication. *N. Engl. J. Med.* **319**: 673–677.

44. Giannini, A.J., Miller, N.S., Loiselle, R.H. and Turner, C.E. (1993) Cocaine-associated violence and relationship to route of administration. *J. Subst. Abuse Treat.* **10**: 67–69.

45. Marzuk, P.M., Tardiff, K., Smyth, D., Stajic, M. and Leon, A.C. (1992) Cocaine use, risk taking and fatal Russian roulette. *J. Am. Med. Assoc.* **267**: 2635–2637.

6

Amphetamines and ecstasy

Bond cursed himself for an impulse that earlier in the day would have seemed unthinkable. Champagne and Benzedrine (amphetamine) – never again.

Ian Fleming, 'Moonraker', 1955.

Illustrated in Figure 6.1 is the wide range of amphetamine derivatives that have been, and still are, abused. Amphetamine itself has been abused since the 1930s but the first derivative to gain acceptance on the street was 3,4-methylenedioxyamphetamine (MDA), known at the time as the 'love drug' because it purportedly dispelled feelings of hate or anger and encouraged emotional closeness between users. MDA abuse began in the USA in the mid-1960s but the drug was declared illegal in 1970. However, a large number of other amphetamine derivatives were introduced during this period and the banning of MDA merely opened the door to related drugs such as MDMA (3,4-methylenedioxymethamphetamine or ecstasy). DOM is an example of an especially hallucinogenic derivative, while methamphetamine is highly stimulatory. MDMA itself seems to have particularly prominent effects on central 5-hydroxytryptamine (5HT) neurones. This may explain why MDMA intoxication seems to involve an overly emotional element. The drug also has a low hallucinogenic potential with less stimulatory effect than amphetamine.

Other related drugs with less potent sympathomimetic effects and less abuse potential, such as phentermine, are still used as appetite suppressants in the treatment of obesity. Another derivative, methylphenidate, is used to treat attention deficit hyperactivity disorder in children.

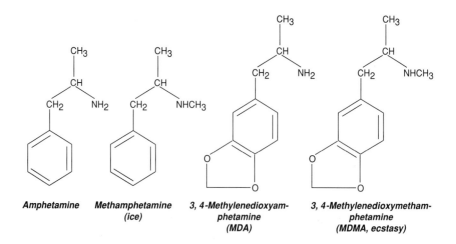

Figure 6.1 Amphetamine and some of its chemical derivatives.
Amphetamine is a racemic mixture of dextro- and laevo-rotatory
amphetamine. D-Amphetamine (dexamphetamine) is the most active
and is the form used therapeutically. Many other amphetamine
derivatives are abused: 3,4-dimethoxymethylamphetamine (DOM or STP);
3,4-methylenedioxyethamphetamine (MDEA or 'Eve');
2-methoxy-3,4-methylenedioxyamphetamine (MMDA);
L-acetyl-3,4-methylenedioxyphenylisoprenaline hydrochloride;
DMA; MDE; MEDA; POM; TMA.

AMPHETAMINE

History

Amphetamine was first synthesised in 1887 and has since been used to
treat a range of medical conditions; some of these are listed in Table
6.1. Amphetamine use proliferated in the 1930s when it was found to
have similar, although more potent, effects to the widely used drug
ephedrine. Ephedrine was extracted from plants and so supplies were
limited and expensive.

Vast quantities of amphetamine were synthesised and issued to
troops and workers during World War II for use as a stimulant during
periods of strenuous activity. Amphetamine was also widely used to treat
comparatively trivial conditions such as rhinitis. Together, these two
factors played a large part in facilitating the early rise of amphetamine
abuse; the population could obtain amphetamine easily and experiment
freely with its psychoactive effects. The drug is known on the street as
'speed', 'whiz' or 'uppers'.

Table 6.1 Therapeutic uses of amphetamine

Historical uses
- Depression
- Anxiety, lethargy and other 'personality' disorders
- Analeptic in barbiturate poisoning
- Appetite suppressant
- Parkinsonism
- Nasal decongestant
- Stimulant for troops and factory workers in wartime
- Nocturnal enuresis

Modern uses of dexamphetamine
- Narcolepsy and other hypersomnic states
- Attention deficit hyperactivity disorder in children
- 'Space sickness', usually in association with hyoscine or an antihistamine

Effects sought

The social abuser seeks the mental and physical stimulation which amphetamine may produce. The individual typically becomes alert, full of self-confidence, happy and talkative; he or she may also feel energetic, strong, impulsive and have increased stamina. This usually lasts up to four hours and as the effects begin to wear off may be succeeded by a period of restlessness, anxiety, fatigue, disinterest or tiredness.

Larger initial doses can provoke an exhilarating euphoria and feelings of great mental power but may also be associated with more intense negative feelings afterwards, such as depression and lethargy (a 'crash'). Regular users develop tolerance such that progressively greater doses are needed with time.

Some abusers seek the stimulating properties of amphetamine for other purposes. Students may use the drug to decrease tiredness, enabling revision for long periods of time. Those in monotonous occupations may abuse amphetamine in the workplace and sportsmen claim that amphetamine enables them to train for longer periods of time.

Administration

Amphetamine may be taken orally, via nasal inhalation or by injection. It is occasionally smoked. Amphetamine is a basic drug and the duration of its effects can be increased by the administration of sodium bicarbonate (baking soda) or any other substance which alkalinises the urine. Alkaline urine favours the formation of the non-ionised form of amphetamine which is much more readily reabsorbed into the

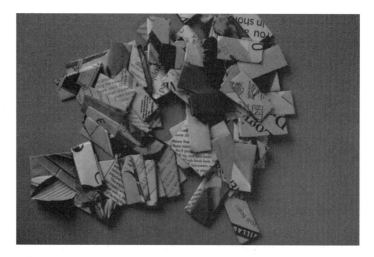

Figure 6.2 'Wraps' of amphetamine powder.

bloodstream from urine. Bicarbonate therefore effectively delays the excretion of amphetamine. Similarly, abusers may use vitamin C, cranberry juice or ammonium chloride to terminate the effects of amphetamine more abruptly when required. It is usually supplied as a white or off-white powder in small card or paper 'wraps' (Figure 6.2).

Pharmacokinetics and pharmacology

Amphetamine is a sympathomimetic agent which principally causes the release of amines from central and peripheral neurones. The main neurotransmitters involved are noradrenaline, dopamine and 5-HT. The detailed pharmacology of many of the amphetamine-related drugs remains to be investigated but most have fewer peripheral actions than amphetamine itself.

The half-lives of both laevo- and dextro-rotatory amphetamine are approximately 12 to 13 hours. The metabolic fate of amphetamine is partly determined by urinary pH, but deamination, N-hydroxylation, aromatic p-hydroxylation and conjugation all occur to varying extents. When urinary pH is unregulated, about 15 per cent of each dose is excreted as unchanged drug [1].

Adverse effects

The onset of amphetamine effects is often heralded by a range of adrenergic 'fight-or-flight' actions, such as sweating and tachycardia; initial side effects can also include nausea, headache and abdominal cramps. These effects may be short-lived or more persistent. A detailed list of adverse reactions is given in Table 6.2. Note that many of the acute, serious adverse effects are inter-related; this is discussed more fully below under ecstasy. Amphetamine will usually only cause rhabdomyolysis and sequelae as a consequence of heavy intravenous use and/or overdose. Unlike ecstasy, the reaction is less commonly linked to overexercise in a hot environment; this may be because amphetamine has a reduced interaction with 5-HT in the brain.

Most psychoactive drugs will occasionally produce unpleasant psychotomimetic effects; these are probably determined by the expectations of the user, their frame of mind at the time and the surroundings. Amphetamine is no exception; extreme anxiety, frightening hallucinations or panic reactions may occur and many of these responses seem to involve paranoid delusions. True psychosis may develop after single or repeated use and can be a long-term problem. It has been suggested that the population most at risk may be those with a predisposition to mental illness.

Although amphetamine does not produce physical dependence there is often a short-lived craving for the drug after cessation of chronic use. This usually responds to simple anti-anxiety management; a withdrawal scheme involving tapered amphetamine dosage is rarely required. Abstinence from amphetamine has been encouraged by the use of a short course of desipramine [2]. However, this treatment has been associated with a 'jitters' reaction which may encourage a return to stimulant abuse because it resembles the euphoria experienced with stimulant drugs [3, 4]. Consequently, fluoxetine has been proposed as a better tolerated alternative and reported to be effective in preventing relapse in two very small studies [4, 5]. An antidepressant may also be needed in the longer term to counteract the depression which is a common finding in those who have abused amphetamine chronically.

METHAMPHETAMINE

History

Methamphetamine has been abused episodically in the past but relatively recently a different form of the drug has appeared in the USA and concern has been expressed that its use may spread rapidly [6]. Just as 'crack' represents a highly purified form of cocaine, 'ice' is a very pure form of methamphetamine which first came to light in Hawaii in the mid-1980s. It is thought that the synthesis procedure allows crystallisation of the drug into tiny colourless spindle shapes which resemble ice crystals, hence the street name. However, the exact preparative process remains unknown. Other street names include 'crystal', 'crank' and 'meth'. The main centres for production appear to be in Southeast Asia and the drug has been popular in Japan. As yet only small-scale abuse has been identified in the UK.

Administration

'Ice' is vaporised, often in a glass tube, and the vapour inhaled to produce a long-lasting 'high' of some 10 to 12 hours. Furthermore, the same sample of drug can be reheated several times and still produce the desired effect because it has a high melting point and is stable to thermal decomposition. The drug is not usually smoked with tobacco because the availability of methamphetamine is thereby greatly reduced [7].

Pharmacokinetics

The half-life following inhalation of methamphetamine vapour has been estimated at an average of 11.7 hours, although a half-life of 10.2 hours was obtained following oral administration [7]. This value is heavily determined by the pH of urine. Aromatic hydroxylation, N-dealkylation and deamination occur in the liver followed by renal elimination. About one-third of a dose is excreted unchanged in urine.

Adverse effects

Relatively little is known about the problems that may be associated with abuse of 'ice'. Some reports suggest that it is highly addictive and that abusers may become violent under the influence of the drug [8]. Methamphetamine has more pronounced stimulatory effects on the central nervous system (CNS) than amphetamine and less potent peripheral actions. However, judgement is impaired and abusers may become restless and agitated; high doses can produce psychotic reactions characterised by hallucinations, paranoia and mania. Post-abuse 'crashes' can also be particularly intense. The drug is known to destroy dopaminergic and serotonergic neurones in the CNS. Other acute and chronic adverse reactions are similar to those experienced after use of amphetamine.

ECSTASY

History

MDMA has a variety of street names including 'Adam', 'XTC', 'M' and 'AKA'. However, it is usually known as 'ecstasy' or 'E'. Some tablets are known by particular names according to the motif embossed upon them (e.g. 'doves'), or their colour (e.g. 'strawberries'). It was first synthesised by E. Merck Pharmaceuticals in 1914 and investigated as an appetite suppressant. However, it was not until MDA was declared an illegal drug in the USA in 1970 that MDMA became widely available. In the 1970s, MDMA was used legally by US psychotherapists to aid counselling [9], particularly in the field of disturbed interpersonal relationships, such as marriage guidance. MDMA was claimed to promote emotional harmony and to reduce enmity. Some therapists still use the drug for this purpose [9]. By 1985, street abuse had reached such heights in the USA that ecstasy was declared an illegal substance. In the UK, the legislature was one step ahead of the illicit manufacturers; all amphetamine-related compounds (including MDMA) were classified as illegal substances under an amendment to the Misuse of Drugs Act as early as 1977.

Effects sought [10]

In the UK, ecstasy has been available in reasonable quantities since the late 1980s. The drug is both synthesised within the UK and imported. Users seek a state of tranquil euphoria in which there is high degree of emotional empathy between associates, greater insight into personal problems and an expanded mental perspective. Abusers feel 'at peace with the world' and aggressive and violent feelings are suppressed. Those under the influence of the drug feel benevolent, less defensive and more interested in interacting with others. The hallucinogenic potential is relatively low, but perceptions may be enhanced. There is often a subjectively altered sense of time. Ecstasy also has amphetamine-like stimulant properties, seeming to give abusers boundless energy although these effects are less potent than those of amphetamine itself.

Although initially associated with the growth of the 'acid house' music scene, in Britain today the use of ecstasy is more intimately associated with the 'rave' culture in which young people, largely between the ages of 16 and 25, gather in night clubs or more secluded 'private' parties and dance through the night to rave music. The term 'rave' is somewhat defunct as a descriptive term at street level but might be used generically to describe a wide range of repetitive musical styles, often with minimal lyrics, which encourage long periods of dancing. Ecstasy can provide the stamina to dance for lengthy periods but this is also the basic cause of some of the more serious side-effects.

Administration

Ecstasy is taken orally, usually in the form of white or off-white tablets which are often embossed and/or scored. These are illustrated in Figures 6.3 and 6.4. Capsules are occasionally seen. A typical dose for a first-time user would be 75 to 100 mg but because of the development of tolerance the dose needs to be gradually increased to achieve the same effect if taken regularly. However, there is no evidence of physical dependence. A regular user might take up to 200 mg as a single dose followed by a smaller booster dose several hours later in order to maintain the intoxication.

Some abusers use ecstasy in association with other drugs. Nitrites, LSD and amphetamine are commonly used concurrently. Users may also employ a variety of preparations to make the aftermath of an ecstasy experience more tolerable. This is called 'coming down'. Preparations used include Vicks VapoRub or Sinex, the caffeine-rich herbal product guarana, and fluoxetine. Some users, aware of the potential 5-HT-depleting properties of ecstasy (see below), may take 'smart drug' drinks containing 5-HT precursors in an attempt to prevent any CNS damage. Smart drugs are discussed in Chapter 18.

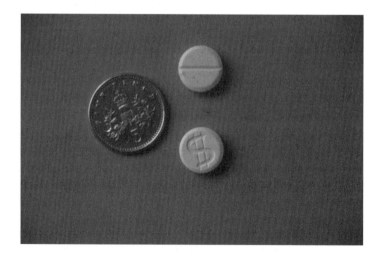

Figure 6.3   Ecstasy tablets. These tablets are well made.

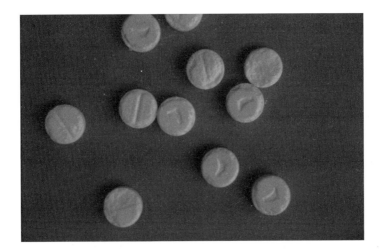

Figure 6.4 Ecstasy tablets. This is a more typical appearance for
ecstasy. The tablets have been pressed inexpertly, such that some have split or
crumbled. The surface texture is rough and similar to 'extra strong mints'.
The dove symbol is also very typical.

It is clear that many ecstasy tablets do not contain pure ecstasy.
A variety of patterns have emerged [11–13]:

- A small proportion of tablets contain no psychoactive drugs at all.
- Most tablets contain ecstasy together with a variety of adulterants
  including caffeine, paracetamol, amphetamine, methamphetamine,
  MDEA, ephedrine, selegiline and ketamine.
- Some tablets contain ecstasy alone.
- Other tablets contain a psychoactive substitute for ecstasy, e.g. keta-
  mine, MDEA, MDA or any one of the bewildering array of
  amphetamine derivatives which exist.

This lack of purity makes it difficult to identify the substance abused
and to treat any adverse effects.

Pharmacokinetics

The average half-life of ecstasy is 7.6 hours [14]. Approximately two-
thirds of a dose is eliminated unchanged in the urine [15]. About 7 per
cent of a dose is excreted as MDA which is also psychoactive.

Adverse effects

Whenever a novel substance of abuse appears, the immediate concern
of non-users is the toxicity potential. In the case of ecstasy this has
been of particular concern because until recently it had been 'marketed'

as a 'clean' drug (i.e. no side-effects). Broadly speaking it appears to have a similar side-effect profile to amphetamine in most respects (see Table 6.2) but few data are available. Many abusers take the drug intermittently, use other drugs concomitantly or in-between times and have only vague ideas of the doses taken. To further complicate the picture, many samples are not pure but contain a range of excipients from harmless bulking agents to other street drugs. Consequently, the abuser is most unlikely to know exactly what he or she has taken.

As with amphetamine, the desired effects are heralded by a 'fight-or-flight' type of reaction and some individuals feel sick or have a headache. Bruxism (grinding of the teeth) or trismus (uncomfortable rigidity of the jaw muscles) are more common with ecstasy than with amphetamine.

Many of the more severe adverse effects of ecstasy are believed to be linked in aetiology (see Figure 6.5). The stimulant properties of the drug can lead individuals to overexercise on the dance floor. This may lead simply to dehydration or later exhaustion but, depending on the level of activity, can progress to rhabdomyolysis (skeletal muscle breakdown) and/or hyperpyrexia. Hyperpyrexia may trigger convulsions or collapse and further fuels the process of rhabdomyolysis. This in turn may result in acute renal failure, either via muscle breakdown products accumulating in the kidney tubules or via disseminated intravascular coagulation. Rhabdomyolysis is not always easy to diagnose because although it often produces muscle pain, swelling and tenderness, many patients are asymptomatic.

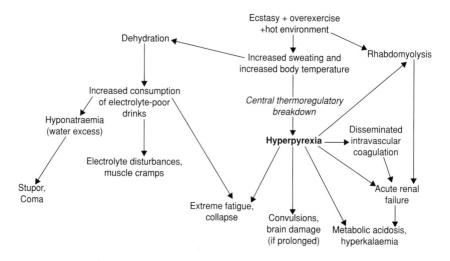

Figure 6.5 Simplified aetiological relationship between some of the more serious adverse effects of ecstasy. These effects have also been described with other amphetamine derivatives.

Hyperpyrexia seems to play an important role in the development of many aspects of severe ecstasy toxicity. It is known that the drug affects the production of 5-HT in the brain of animals, so disruption of 5-HT transmission in the human hypothalamus may incapacitate central thermoregulatory control in some way. This pattern of adverse effects can occur with other amphetamine-related drugs but in the UK has been described most consistently with ecstasy, probably because of the close association between ecstasy and dance music (i.e. high levels of physical activity). The chain of events is not necessarily linked to the dose although higher doses probably increase the risk. First-time users are just as vulnerable as those who abuse the drug regularly.

In the USA, where ecstasy does not tend to be abused in this milieu, hyperpyrexia associated adverse effects are more rarely reported. In the UK, many fatalities have been reported. The hyperpyrexia has been treated with dantrolene.

The risks of hyperpyrexia-related death or serious injury can be reduced by encouraging users to following some straightforward advice, including:

■ Avoid dancing for prolonged periods of time. Take regular rests and relax in a cool place for a while. Many nightclub owners and hosts of rave events provide 'chill out' areas for this purpose.
■ Drink plenty of fluid to reduce dehydration but avoid overhydration. Taking electrolyte replacement solutions is to be preferred.
■ Wear light, loose clothes.

An increasingly reported problem is that of hyponatraemia [16–20]. This occurs when the subject becomes very thirsty and drinks excessive quantities of salt-poor fluids. This polydipsia could be due simply to becoming hot whilst taking exercise (dancing) and following the standard advice to drink plenty of fluid when taking ecstasy. This can lead to severe water intoxication and hyponatraemia. However, it has also been suggested that ecstasy can cause the syndrome of inappropriate secretion of antidiuretic hormone (SIADH) [16–18] but this has been disputed [21, 22]. Whatever the precise mechanism of hyponatraemia the effects of it can be severe. Agitation, variable consciousness, dystonias, cerebral oedema, convulsions and coma are notable sequelae. Deaths have occurred.

Animal studies have shown that ecstasy is neurotoxic [23, 24]. In various mammals, destruction of central 5-HT neurones and decreased synthesis of 5-HT has been demonstrated. Primates appear to be even more sensitive to this effect than rats, since the effects may be permanent. However, it is not clear whether these changes will occur in man,

Table 6.2 Potential side-effects of amphetamine and ecstasy-related drugs

Minor adverse effects

Relatively common and generally short-lived reactions, which occur shortly after taking a dose:

- Mydriasis, photophobia
- Headache
- Anorexia, nausea, dry mouth, abdominal cramps, diarrhoea
- Sweating, tachypnoea, tachycardia, palpitations, tremor ('fight-or-flight' reaction)
- Bruxism (grinding of the teeth)
- Trismus (uncomfortable rigidity of the jaw muscles)
- Gait disturbance, ataxia

Serious acute adverse effects

These reactions are not common:

- Unpleasant hallucinations, severe anxiety, agitation, panic attacks, paranoia
- Hypertension, especially with amphetamine
- Cardiac arrhythmias [30, 13]
- Cardiomyopathy [30–32]
- Intracerebral haemorrhage [33]
- Severe central chest pain (probably due to intercostal muscle spasm) [34]
- Severe abdominal cramps
- Accidental death or injury while in intoxicated state, e.g.
  road traffic accidents [35, 30]
  aspiration of vomit [36]
- Urinary retention; one case reported after a very large dose of ecstasy [37]

In certain circumstances*

- Over-exertion, dehydration, collapse
- Hyperpyrexia
- Convulsions (with or without hyperpyrexia or history of epilepsy) [40, 41]
- Rhabdomyolysis
- Disseminated intravascular coagulation, cerebrovascular accidents
- Acute renal failure, metabolic acidosis
- Polydipsia, hyponatraemia and stupor [42, 43, 13]

Delayed reactions to exposure

These side-effects occur after exposure to amphetamines:

- Chronic exhaustion, fatigue, muscular aches (may persist for several days after a single dose)
- Jaundice, hepatotoxicity [35, 44, 45, 13]
- Weight loss (associated with repeated use and due to increased amount of exercise while intoxicated and the anorexic effects of amphetamines)
- 'Flashbacks' (repeatedly experiencing a (usually) unpleasant 'trip' some time after the original event [46])
- Insomnia (may be persistent)
- Depression (associated with withdrawal; usually brief after short-term use but may be chronic following discontinuation of a long-term habit)
- Psychosis (may be an acute short-lived reaction or a more persistent problem [46, 47])

*Many of these effects have a related aetiology (see Figure 6.2 and text). In ecstasy users, overexercise in a hot environment seems to be an important aetiological factor [35, 38]; in amphetamine users, high doses are more likely to be the cause [39].

whether they are reversible or not, or even if they are important. Physically, animals with ecstasy-induced neurological changes were indistinguishable from controls.

When damaged nerve tissue regrows after exposure to ecstasy in animals, it does so slowly. It is also incomplete. The axons generated do not make the same connections to adjacent nerves as their predecessors [25]. The implications of this drug-induced 're-wiring' are unclear. At high doses, ecstasy also damages dopaminergic neurones.

If ecstasy causes long-lasting damage to central 5-HT pathways in humans, drug abuse might result in a range of chronic disorders. For example, serotonergic neurones are prevalent in areas of the brain connected with emotions and many antidepressant drugs enhance their effects. In addition, CNS turnover of this neurotransmitter is reduced in those suffering from depression. Ecstasy, like amphetamine, can also trigger temporary or persistent psychosis. The long-term legacy of ecstasy abuse might be a tendency towards endogenous depression or other mood disorder. Lethargy and depression after the effects of ecstasy have worn off are quite common reactions. This might be a psychological response in certain individuals who feel so content and cheerful during an ecstasy trip that 'real life' seems very unsatisfactory by comparison. On the other hand, it might equally be due to an ecstasy-induced depletion of central 5-HT. At the time of writing it is not known whether ecstasy can cause serotonergic neurone damage in humans, although the concentration of serotonin metabolites in cerebrospinal fluid are decreased for weeks after exposure to ecstasy and this could be due to increased destruction of serotonergic nerve tissue [26]. Nerve destruction has been observed in all other mammalian species studied.

Immunosuppressant properties have been attributed to ecstasy, because abusers seem more likely to contract colds and other minor infections. These effects may be more related to the abuser's lifestyle than to the drug itself. Dancing in a hot, crowded environment is very conducive to the spread of minor infectious diseases and to the development of 'chills' after leaving the gathering.

AMPHETAMINE-RELATED MEDICINES

Diethylpropion, phentermine, methylphenidate and pemoline are all controlled by the Misuse of Drugs Act. Since black market availability of these drugs is limited, street abuse is a comparatively minor problem. The drugs have only mild amphetamine-like properties and so large doses are needed for the purpose of abuse.

Methylphenidate is probably the most widely abused of the prescription amphetamine derivatives. The drug has only weak amphetamine effects when taken orally due to poor bioavailability. However, these drawbacks are overcome when it is abused by the intravenous route. This practice has been reported particularly from the USA. The injection is prepared by crushing tablets and dissolving the drug in water.

Wolf *et al.* described an 'eosinophilic syndrome' in 16 intravenous methylphenidate abusers [27]. This was typically characterised by eosinophilia, fever, musculoskeletal complaints (e.g. arthralgia) and pulmonary symptoms (e.g. pleuritic chest pain, dyspnoea, wheezing). The exact presentation varied quite widely between patients. The reaction may have been at least partly due to tablet excipients.

Retinopathy was described in a series of 12 patients in the USA [28]. Emboli of insoluble tablet excipients were probably responsible (see Chapter 2). Sufficient emboli can wedge in the blood vessels of the lungs to cause pulmonary hypertension and a death has been reported [29]. In a group of 22 intravenous methylphenidate abusers, the average daily dose was 200 mg (range: 40–700 mg) [29]. Abusers, who all had a history of drug abuse, often obtained the drug initially after their children were prescribed the drug for hyperactivity. Later, supplies were maintained by duping a variety of physicians into prescribing it or by altering legitimate prescriptions in their favour.

Several over-the-counter sympathomimetic drugs have amphetamine-like properties and are sometimes abused. Examples include pseudoephedrine and phenylpropanolamine (see Chapter 12).

REFERENCES

1. Dollery, C. (ed.) (1991) Dexamphetamine Sulphate, in *Therapeutic Drugs*, Churchill Livingstone, Edinburgh, pp. D50–D55.
2. Tennant, F.S., Tarver, A., Pumphrey, E. and Seecof, R. (1986) Double-blind comparison of desipramine and placebo for treatment of phencyclidine or amphetamine dependence. *NIDA Res. Monogr.* **67**: 310–317.
3. Weiss, R.D. (1988) Relapse to cocaine abuse after initiating desipramine treatment. *J. Am. Med. Assoc.* **260**: 2545–2546.
4. Polson, R., O'Shea, J.K. and Fleming, P.M. (1992) Fluoxetine in the treatment of illegal drug withdrawal (letter). *Hum. Psychopharmacol.* **7**: 223–224.
5. Polson, R.G., Fleming, P.M. and O'Shea, J.K (1993) Fluoxetine in the treatment of amphetamine dependence. *Hum. Psychopharmacol.* **8**: 55–58.

6. Jaffe, J. (1989) The re-emergence of methamphetamine. *Statement before select committee on narcotics abuse and control, US House of Representatives,* October 24, 1989. Department of Health and Human Services, USA.

7. Cook, C.E. (1991) Pyrolytic characteristics, pharmacokinetics and bioavailability of smoked heroin, cocaine, phencyclidine and methamphetamine. *NIDA Res. Monogr.* **115**: 6–24.

8. News (1990) Crack – yesterday's drug as ice sweeps Hawaii. *Druglink,* **5**: 7.

9. Saunders, N. (1995) *Ecstasy and the Dance Culture.* Nicholas Saunders Publishers, Exeter, pp. 14–15, 124–137.

10. Liester, M.B., Grob, C.S., Bravo, G.L. and Walsh, R.N. (1992) Phenomenology and sequelae of 3,4-methylenedioxymethamphetamine use. *J. Nerv. Ment. Dis.* **180**: 345–352.

11. Wolff, K., Hay, A.W.M., Sherlock, K., Conner, M (1995) Contents of ecstasy (letter). *Lancet,* **346**: 1100–1101.

12. Saunders, N. (1995) *Ecstasy and the Dance Culture.* Nicholas Saunders Publishers, Exeter, pp. 149–50, 161–163.

13. Milroy, C.M., Clark, J.C. and Forrest, A.R.W. (1996) Pathology of deaths associated with 'ecstasy' and 'eve' misuse. *J. Clin. Pathol.* **49**: 149–153.

14. Baselt, R.C. and Cravey, R.H. (1989) *The Disposition of Toxic Drugs and Chemicals in Man,* Yearbook Medical Publications, London, 3rd edn, p. 554.

15. Alrazi, J. and Verebey, K. (1988) MDMA biological disposition in man: MDA is a biotransformation product. *NIDA Res. Monogr.* **90**: 34.

16. Holden, R. and Jackson, M.A. (1996) Near-fatal hyponatraemic coma due to vasopressin oversecretion after 'ecstasy' (3,4-MDMA) (letter). *Lancet,* **347**: 1052.

17. Satchell, S.C. and Connaughton, M. (1994) Inappropriate antidiuretic hormone secretion and extreme rises in serum creatinine kinase following MDMA ingestion. *Br. J. Hosp. Med.* **51**: 495.

18. Matthai, S.M., Davidson, D.C., Sills, J.A. and Alexandrou, S. (1996) Cerebral oedema after ingestion of MDMA ('ecstasy') and unrestricted intake of water (letter). *Br. Med. J.* **312**: 1359.

19. Maxwell, D.L., Pikey, M.I. and Henry, J.A. (1993) Hyponatraemia and catatonic stupor after taking 'ecstasy' (letter). *Br. Med. J.* **307**: 1399.

20. Kessel, B. (1994) Hyponatraemia after ingestion of 'ecstasy'. *Br. Med. J.* **308**: 414.

21. Cook, T.M. (1996) Cerebral oedema after MDMA ('ecstasy') and unrestricted water intake (letter). *Br. Med. J.* **313**: 689.

22. Wilkins, B. (1996) Hyponatraemia must be treated with low water input (letter). *Br. Med. J.* **313**: 689–690.

23. Ricaurte, G., Bryan, G., Strauss, L., Seiden, L. and Schuster, C. (1985) Hallucinogenic amphetamine selectively destroys brain serotonin nerve terminals. *Science,* **229**: 986–988.

24. Steele, T.D., McCann, U.D. and Ricaurte, G.A. (1994) 3,4-methylene-dioxymethamphetamine (MDMA, ecstasy): pharmacology and toxicology in animals and humans. *Addiction*, **89**: 539–551.

25. Fischer, C., Hatzidimitriou, G., Wlos, J., Katz, J. and Ricaurte, G. (1995) Reorganisation of ascending 5-HT axon projections in animals previously exposed to the recreational drug (±)3,4-methylenedioxymethamphetamine (MDMA, 'Ecstasy'). *J. Neurosci.* **15**: 5476–5485.

26. McCann, U.D., Ridenour, A., Shaham, Y. and Ricaurte, G.A. (1994) Serotonergic neurotoxicity after (±)3,4-methylenedioxymethamphetamine (MDMA, 'Ecstasy'): a controlled study in humans. *Neuropsychopharmacol.* **10**: 129–138.

27. Wolf, J., Fein, A. and Fehrenbacher, L. (1978) Eosinophilic syndrome with methylphenidate abuse. *Ann. Intern. Med.* **89**: 224–225.

28. Gunby, P. (1979) Methylphenidate abuse produces retinopathy. *J. Am. Med. Assoc.* **241**: 546.

29. Parran (Jr), T.V. and Jasinski, D.R. (1991) Intravenous methylphenidate abuse – Prototype for prescription drug abuse. *Arch. Intern. Med.* **151**: 781–783.

30. Dowling, G.P., McDonough, E.T. and Bost, R.O. (1987) Eve and Ecstasy a report of five deaths associated with the use of MDEA and MDMA. *J. Am. Med. Assoc.* **257**: 1615–1617.

31. Hong, R., Matsuyama, E. and Nur, K. (1991) Cardiomyopathy associated with the smoking of crystal methamphetamine. *J. Am. Med. Assoc.* **265**: 1152–1154.

32. Call, T.D., Hartneck, J., Dickinson, W.A., Hartman, C.W. and Bartel, A.G. (1982) Acute cardiomyopathy secondary to intravenous amphetamine abuse. *Ann. Intern. Med.* **97**: 559–560.

33. Harries, D.P. and de Silva, R.N. (1992) Ecstasy and intracerebral haemorrhage. *Scott. Med. J.* **370**: 150–152.

34. Rittoo, D., Rittoo, D.B. and Rittoo, D. (1992) Misuse of ecstasy (letter). *Br. Med. J.* **305**: 309–310.

35. Henry, J.A., Jeffreys, K.J. and Dawling, S. (1992) Toxicity and deaths from 3,4-methylenedioxymethamphetamine ('ecstasy'). *Lancet*, **340**: 384–387.

36. Forrest, A.R.W., Galloway, J.H., Marsh, I.D., Strachan, G.A. and Clark, J.C. (1994) A fatal overdose with 3,4-methylenedioxymethamphetamine derivatives. *Forensic Sci. Int.* **64**: 57–59.

37. Bryden, A.A., Rothwell, P.J.N. and O'Reilly, P.H. (1995) Urinary retention with misuse of ecstasy (Drug Points). *Br. Med. J.* **310**: 504.

38. Henry, J.A. (1992) Ecstasy and the dance of death. *Br. Med. J.* **305**: 5–6.

39. Ginsberg, M.D., Hertzman, M. and Schmidt-Nowara, W.W. (1970) Amphetamine intoxication with coagulopathy, hyperthermia, and reversible renal failure. *Ann. Intern. Med.* **73**: 81–85.

40. Alldredge, B.K., Lowenstein, D.H. and Simon, R.P. (1989) Seizures associated with recreational drug abuse. *Neurology*, **39**: 1037–1039.

41. Sawyer, J. and Stephens, W.P. (1992) Misuse of ecstasy (letter). *Br. Med. J.* **305**: 310.
42. Maxwell, D.L., Polkey, M.I. and Henry, J.A. (1993) Hyponatraemia and catatonic stupor after taking ecstasy. *Br. Med. J.* **307**: 1399.
43. Kessel, B. (1994) Hyponatraemia after ingestion of ecstasy (letter). *Br. Med. J.* **308**: 414.
44. Shearman, J.D., Chapman, R.W.G., Satsangi, J., Ryley, N.G. and Weatherhead, S. (1992) Misuse of ecstasy (letter). *Br. Med. J.* **305**: 309.
45. Gorard, D.A., Davies, S.E. and Clark, M.L. (1992) Misuse of ecstasy (letter). *Br. Med. J.* **305**: 309.
46. Creighton, F.J., Black, D.L. and Hyde, C.E. (1991) Ecstasy psychosis and flashbacks *Br. J. Psychiatr.* **159**: 713–715.
47. McGuire, P. and Fahy, T. (1991) Chronic paranoid psychosis after misuse of MDMA (ecstasy). *Br. Med. J.* **302**: 697.

7

LSD

*When I closed my eyes, an unending series of
colourful, very realistic and fantastic images surged
in upon me. A remarkable feature was the manner
in which all acoustic perceptions (e.g. the noise of a
passing car) were transformed into optical effects,
every sound evoking a corresponding coloured
hallucination constantly changing in shape and
colour like pictures in a kaleidoscope.*
Albert Hofmann, from notes made following
self-administration of LSD, 1943.

HISTORY

LSD has many street names but is most commonly referred to as 'acid'
or 'trips'. It is also known as lysergic acid diethylamide or lysergide, and
was first synthesised by Hofmann and Stoll of Sandoz in 1938. It was
derived from lysergic acid, a non-psychoactive compound found in ergot,
a common fungal contaminant of rye and other cereal crops. The initials
LSD are derived from the German name for the drug: Lyserg Saure
Diethylamid. Following investigation as a 'psychotherapeutic' aid in the
UK and the USA during the 1950s and 1960s [1], illicit use began to
spread rapidly. In 1991 a National Household survey in the USA revealed
that 5.9 per cent of the population had used LSD on at least one occasion [2]. LSD has been an illegal substance in the UK since 1966.

EFFECTS SOUGHT

As with amphetamine derivatives, LSD often produces an initial burst
of adrenaline-like activity characterised by flushing, hypertension, dry
mouth, tachycardia, mydriasis, sweating, tremor etc. These effects usually

begin within ten minutes of taking an oral dose and may persist through the rest of the experience. Sometimes the abuser may feel nauseous at the outset. As this initial stage progresses and within 30 to 60 minutes of administration, the individual may begin to experience euphoria which is usually accompanied or followed by a range of 'psychedelic' effects (the 'trip'). These effects include:

- emotional lability;
- time distortions, including perceptions of rapid ageing (of self or others);
- visual and auditory illusions (colours and sound may be enhanced or magnified; real images may assume unusual colours or patterns);
- synaesthesia (a mixing of sensory input, so that the abuser may 'see' sounds or smells, and 'hear' or 'feel' colours, etc.);
- the events often have mystic, religious or philosophical overtones. The individual may become depersonalised and detached from reality, become 'at peace with the world' or undergo 'out-of-the-body' experiences.

During the recovery period, as the effects of an LSD dose are beginning to wear off, the subject may experience episodes of normality alternating with psychedelic effects.

Most of the mind-altering properties of LSD involve distortion or misinterpretation of real sensory stimuli (i.e. illusions) rather than completely false perceptions without any sensory stimulus (hallucinations) although true hallucinations can occur. LSD also causes delusions (false beliefs) such as believing one to be invincible or able to fly. Consequently, although LSD is typically described as an hallucinogenic drug, this is rather misleading. Alternative descriptions that can be used are: illusionogenic or illusogenic (illusion producing) and psychedelic (producing an expansion of the mind and widening of perception).

ADMINISTRATION

LSD is nearly always administered orally, although nasal inhalation, injection, smoking and conjunctival instillation have been reported [3]. The dose required is small, usually between 50 and 200 micrograms, and is usually taken as small pieces of paper which have been impregnated with the drug (Figure 7.1). Tiny tablets or microdots are occasionally seen (Figure 7.2). The smallest doses are taken by the inexperienced; sometimes as little as 20 micrograms. Tablets, gelatin squares, sugar cubes, capsules or liquid preparations are rarely seen. Paper squares are often adorned with brightly coloured designs or motifs such as

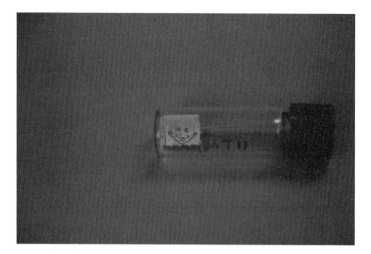

Figure 7.1 LSD blotter (actual size 8 mm^2). A drop of LSD solution is impregnated onto blotting paper with a printed design.

animals, geometric shapes, signs of the zodiac or cartoon characters. The drug is odourless, colourless and tasteless.

There have been a number of 'scares' in recent years that LSD might be given to unsuspecting schoolchildren *en masse* by drug dealers in the form of skin transfers 'to get them hooked'. There is no evidence that LSD is absorbed through normal, intact human skin in amounts sufficient to cause intoxication. It is also most unlikely that drug dealers would give away supplies of LSD and because the drug is known not to cause physical dependence the idea seems fanciful. Unfortunately, many parents have been unnecessarily alarmed by hoaxes of this kind which have been reported from the USA, Canada, Germany and the UK. All have been without foundation [4, 5].

PHARMACOKINETICS AND PHARMACOLOGY

The mechanism of action of the drug is unclear. It is thought to interact with both serotonergic and dopaminergic systems in the central nervous system but serotonergic effects probably predominate. The psychedelic effects of LSD usually take 30 to 90 minutes to begin after an oral dose and they last three to 12 hours, depending on the dose and the individual. (The average duration is six to eight hours). The half-life is about eight hours [6] and the main route of elimination is via the liver. Hydroxylation and conjugation is followed by excretion into bile [7].

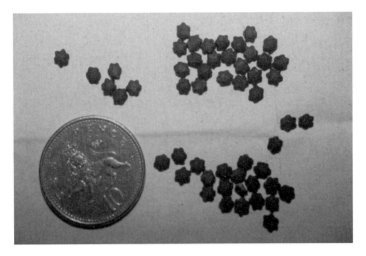

Figure 7.2 LSD microdots. Small tablets which may be round or shaped.

ADVERSE EFFECTS

Apart from the adrenergic-like actions already mentioned, exhaustion, headaches, muscular weakness and inability to concentrate are quite common. Most adverse effects are related to the mind-altering properties of the drug. Bad 'trips' may involve prolonged panic attacks, general dysphoria, acute depression or frightening illusions. It has been advocated that pharmacological intervention should be avoided in patients presenting with distressing experiences of this kind and that those affected should be 'talked down' in a quiet place. In extreme situations, low dose intramuscular haloperidol or lorazepam have been used [8]. Table 7.1 summarises the adverse effects.

Unpleasant experiences were categorised in one US study of 107 LSD users [9]. Results were as follows: terror, 39 per cent; crawling insects or animals, 18 per cent; Satan's face appearing, 18 per cent; ageing of others' faces, 12 per cent; delusion of insanity, 5 per cent.

LSD abusers tend to remain conscious and relatively communicative when prompted, even at the height of intoxication.

Psychedelic effects occasionally result in curious injuries or acts of violence (against self or others) while in the intoxicated state. In the study by Schwartz [9], 23 LSD users from a total of 107 declared that they or a close friend had been involved in a serious accident or had made a suicide attempt whilst under the influence of LSD. Delusions of being able to fly or of being invincible can also have serious consequences.

Table 7.1 Adverse effects of LSD

Common acute reactions
- Adrenergic 'fight or flight' effects (tachycardia, flushing, dry mouth, sweating etc.)
- Exhaustion, tiredness, weakness
- Inability to concentrate, anxiety, dysphoria, panic, frightening illusions, delusions or hallucinations, psychosis
- Self-harm, accidents or violence while intoxicated

Rare acute reactions
- Ataxia, convulsions
- Paraesthesiae
- Hyperpyrexia, neuroleptic malignant syndrome (one case report attributed to LSD plus alcohol [10])

Post-exposure reactions
- 'Flashbacks'
- Depression, feelings of isolation, tiredness, delirium

Psychosis can develop after a single dose and may become a chronic problem. As with amphetamines, it is not clear whether this represents a true drug-induced condition or the unmasking of a latent mental illness. Psychosis generally occurs after chronic use of LSD and in this respect differs from amphetamine-induced psychosis which can occur after a single dose. Acute depression, loneliness, tiredness or delirium can occur shortly after the effects of LSD have worn off, but is usually short-lived.

'Flashbacks' can also be a persistent problem [5]. These phenomena are psychedelic effects experienced long after the drug has been eliminated from the body. They are more likely to occur in those who use the drug regularly and are generally not reported by those who use LSD on a small number of occasions. Sometimes they are referred to by the more grandiose title of 'post-hallucinogen perceptual disorder'. In one study [9] 64 per cent of 107 chronic users reported flashbacks but only 16 per cent found these persistent or worrying. Flashbacks can develop a few days after LSD intoxication or up to one year later and involve any aspect of a previous 'trip'. They may continue for years after exposure but tend to diminish in intensity and frequency with time. Common components of flashbacks are the illusion that stationary objects are moving, haloes, the sudden appearance of bright patterns, time distortions and other visual or auditory hallucinations and illusions. Sometimes flashbacks are brought on by later abuse of other drugs (e.g. alcohol, cannabis) or by physical or emotional stress. Haloperidol may help to suppress their reappearance.

LSD overdose is reported infrequently. Features on presentation may include mydriasis, hypertension, tachycardia, respiratory arrest, convulsions, hyperpyrexia or coma. Physical dependence does not occur and psychological dependence is uncommon, short-lived and often responds to standard antianxiety measures. Tolerance may occur in the chronic abuser, but a few days' abstinence will restore full central nervous system sensitivity to the drug.

REFERENCES

1. Dyer, C. (1995) Patients given LSD may be able to claim compensation (news). *Br. Med. J.* **311**: 1185–1186.
2. Anon. (1995) LSD (Lysergic Acid Diethylamide). *NIDA Capsule (CAP 39)*, National Institute on Drug Abuse, USA, 1–4.
3. Kulig, K. (1990) LSD. *Emerg. Med. Clin. N. Am.* **8**: 551–558.
4. Babin, L. (October 1988) Blue Star LSD: A Psychedelic Hoax. *R. Can. Mounted Police Bull.* 23–25.
5. Schwartz, R.H. (1995) LSD: Its rise, fall, and renewed popularity among high school students. *Pediatr. Clin. N. Am.* **42** (2): 403–413.
6. Aghajanian, G.K. and Bing, O.H.C. (1964) Persistence of lysergic acid diethylamide in the plasma of human subjects. *Clin. Pharmacol. Ther.* **5**: 611–614.
7. Renkel, M. (1957) Pharmacodynamics of LSD and mescaline. *J. Nerv. Ment. Dis.* **125**: 424–427.
8. Miller, P.L., Gay, G.R., Ferris, K.C. and Anderson, S. (1992) Treatment of acute, adverse psychedelic reactions: 'I've tripped and I can't get down'. *J. Psychoactive Drugs*, **24**: 277–279.
9. Schwartz, R.H. (1987) LSD: Patterns of use by chemically dependent adolescents. *J. Pediatr.* **111**: 936–938.
10. Bakheit, A.M.O., Behan, P.O., Prach, A.T., Rittey, C.D. and Scott, A.J. (1990) A syndrome identical to the neuroleptic malignant syndrome induced by LSD and alcohol (letter). *Br. J. Addiction Alcohol Other Drugs*, **85**: 150–151.

Phencyclidine

It produces profound analgesia to a degree that even some major surgical procedures may be done without supplemental drugs. It has the decided disadvantage of producing in some patients severe excitement on emergence and severe hallucinatory disturbances.

Description of the first clinical study of phencyclidine use in humans as an anaesthetic (1958) [1].

HISTORY

Phencyclidine (PCP or 'angel dust') was investigated as an intravenous anaesthetic in the 1950s but was withdrawn from the market because it produced unpleasant hallucinations, agitation and delirium in humans. The product was later used as a veterinary anaesthetic but is no longer available. Abuse has not been a major problem in the UK and even in the USA, where phencyclidine was once of serious concern, abuse now appears to be much less common and more localised (e.g. Washington DC). A US study in 1994 reported that 1.6 per cent of senior pupils at high school had used phencyclidine compared with 7 per cent in 1979 [2]. A large number of derivatives has been developed illicitly but none of these has gained widespread acceptance on the street. An example is 1-(1-phenylcyclohexyl)pyrrolidine or PHP; others include PCC, PCE and TCP.

EFFECTS SOUGHT

Abusers seek euphoria, which develops within a few minutes after smoking and is often accompanied by unusual delusions and hallucinations. The acute 'high' lasts some four to six hours but it may take a few days for the effects to wear off completely. Some users find that the drug gives them feelings of power and invulnerability.

ADMINISTRATION

Phencyclidine is usually smoked, often mixed with leafy material (e.g. tobacco, cannabis), but can also be administered orally, intravenously and by nasal inhalation of dry powder. It has a characteristic bitter taste. In the USA, phencyclidine has been a common adulterant of other illicit drugs because it is cheap and easy to make.

PHARMACOKINETICS AND PHARMACOLOGY

The mode of action of phencyclidine is not understood but it is known to affect a range of central neurotransmitter systems, which probably accounts for the wide variety of side-effects that have been reported (see Table 8.1). The half-life of phencyclidine varies greatly, from seven hours to over three days [3,4]. The drug is eliminated primarily by hydroxylation in the liver followed by kidney excretion. About 10 per cent of circulating phencyclidine is excreted as unchanged drug in the urine.

ADVERSE EFFECTS

Those intoxicated with phencyclidine typically show frequent changes in behaviour and level of alertness [3, 5] (see Table 8.1). As with ketamine, to which it is closely related chemically, much concern has centred on the unusual perceptual distortions, mind-altering and behavioural effects of phencyclidine. Many first-time users find the experience unpleasant and do not use it again. In the USA particularly, these strange dissociative and psychotomimetic effects have resulted in bizarre accidents and acts of self-harm or violence. Phencyclidine-induced psychosis can be peculiarly persistent and may take weeks or even months to dissipate; as with many other drugs of abuse it is unclear whether phencyclidine simply unmasks or exacerbates a tendency to psychosis or causes the illness *de novo* [6].

Phencyclidine is a very lipophilic drug and symptoms of intoxication may sometimes reappear two or three days after the original

Table 8.1 Adverse effects of phencyclidine

Relatively acute problems
- Hypertension (hypertensive crises are rare), tachycardia (common)
- Nausea, vomiting, hypersalivation
- Flushing, sweating, fever, hyperpyrexia (and sequelae)
- Rhabdomyolysis
- Bronchospasm, aspiration pneumonia
- Nystagmus (very common), tremor, slurred speech, dystonias
- Convulsions, catatonia, stupor, coma
- Confusion, dizziness, amnesia
- Euphoria, acute depression, agitation, violence, psychosis, hallucination, delusions, dysphoria, aggression
- Bizarre and dangerous behaviour while intoxicated, sometimes with serious or fatal consequences

Problems connected with chronic abuse
- Psychological and physical dependence
- Chronic anxiety, confusion, depression
- Memory loss, speech difficulties
- Psychosis, various personality changes, 'flashbacks'

exposure when fatty tissues are metabolised and it is released into the circulation again. This delayed reaction, and the central nervous system effects of phencyclidine generally, may be potentiated by barbiturates and opioids (but not benzodiazepines) which should therefore be avoided in those suspected of abuse. Phencyclidine does not cause respiratory depression, despite its anaesthetic properties.

REFERENCES

1. Greifenstein, F.E., DeVault, M., Yoshitake, J. and Gajewski, J.E. (1958) A study of 1-aryl cyclo hexyl amine for anesthesia. *Anesth. Analg.* **37**: 283–294.
2. Anon. (1995) PCP (Phencyclidine). *NIDA Capsule (CAP14)*, National Institute on Drug Abuse, USA, pp. 1–2.
3. Baldridge, E.B. (1990) Phencyclidine. *Emerg. Med. Clin. N. Am.* **8** (3): 541–550.
4. Cook, C.E., Brine, D.R. and Jeffcoat, A.R. (1982) Phencyclidine disposition after intravenous and oral doses. *Clin. Pharmacol. Ther.* **31**: 625–634.
5. Isaacs, S.O., Martin, P. and Washington, J.A. (1986) Phencyclidine (PCP) abuse. *Oral Surg. Oral Med. Oral Pathol.* **61**: 126–129.
6. Wright, H.H., Cole, E.A., Batey, S.R. and Hanna, K. (1988) Phencyclidine-induced psychosis: eight year follow-up of ten cases. *South. Med. J.* **81**: 565–567.

9

Volatile substance abuse

Dr Snow gave that blessed chloroform and the effect was soothing, quieting and delightful beyond measure.
Queen Victoria describing the administration of anaesthetic chloroform in her Journal.

HISTORY

Volatile substance abuse (VSA) can be defined as 'deliberate inhalation of a volatile substance to achieve a change in mental state' [1]. Compulsive abuse of ether and chloroform was known in Victorian England and in Ireland but this was a relatively minor problem compared to the wider abuse of other substances such as opium. It was not until the 1970s that UK mortality data for VSA became available and the problem then began to attract medical and media attention. The number of deaths attributed to VSA gradually increased until 1990 but there has been a decline since then. In 1990, the number of deaths peaked at 151. In 1991 this fell to 122, then 84 in 1992, 71 in 1993 and by 1994 – the latest year for which figures are available – the number of fatalities was 57 [2]. This decline is most welcome but the reasons for it are unknown. It may represent a genuine decrease in use due to recognition of the potential adverse consequences. Alternatively, and more likely, other abusable substances have become more popular [3]. Tobacco and alcohol are readily available. There is evidence for increased use of tobacco amongst teenage girls in particular and certain alcoholic products seem to be marketed with teenagers in mind. Ecstasy, but also cannabis, has become cheaper and more fashionable.

The volatile substances or 'inhalants' are perhaps unique amongst substances of abuse in that the main abusers are children and teenagers: most are between 10 and 18 years old. The majority start when aged between 10 and 14, and, although estimates vary, up to one in 10 secondary school pupils are believed to abuse volatile substances to some degree. However, local statistics show that this figure varies considerably across the country. A survey of 7722 schoolchildren aged 15 or 16 from around the UK was reported in 1996. Self-reported abuse of volatile substances on at least one occasion was described by 21 per cent of girls and 19.7 per cent of boys [3]. In 1992, the Department of Health considered that about 70 per cent of users 'experimented' with the method a small number of times only, 'but that about 1 per cent of secondary school children became long-term users' [4]. This latter population abuse inhalants regularly for more than three months. In the USA, two large studies estimated the extent of VSA amongst school-age teenagers at 7 to 8 per cent and 16.6 per cent, respectively [1]. It is unclear whether VSA encourages abuse of other substances subsequently.

EFFECTS SOUGHT

The first 'rush' or 'buzz' occurs when a relatively high concentration of inhaled substance reaches the brain quickly. This often produces a rapid 'high' or feeling of intense exhilaration. The subsequent effects can appear similar to drunkenness: feeling merry, playful and uninhibited, and sociability is often increased. The emotions prevalent at the time can be heightened. Unlike alcohol, inhalants commonly cause euphoria, hallucinations and perceptual disturbances. The hallucinations can, to some extent, be controlled and sometimes become a group activity.

All these effects appear very quickly – within minutes – but do not last long. However, the experienced (usually chronic) abuser can sustain the desirable effects for several hours by repeating inhalations when the effects of previous exposures begin to wear off.

There may be a subsequent hangover feeling in some users even after a single exposure. This usually takes the form of drowsiness, headache and inability to concentrate.

It is not always easy to understand why a particular child has taken to volatile substance abuse. Undoubtedly the 'naughtiness' and potential danger associated with a behaviour that would shock or anger parents is an attraction for some. Loneliness, boredom, domestic strife or feelings of inadequacy may sometimes be important causes. For others, solvents are simply an easily-obtainable, affordable alternative to the alcohol consumed by older friends and relatives. Inhalants are still more accessible to many teenagers than tobacco. The hallucinations and loss of control experienced can be pleasurable or frightening, but either way can represent an appealing escape from reality.

There is some evidence that abusers are more likely to come from families at the lower end of the socioeconomic scale and that the incidence is greater in inner city areas. Inhalant abusers are also more likely to play truant from school than other children.

ADMINISTRATION

The terms 'glue-sniffing' and 'solvent misuse' only cover part of the problem. Numerous products are involved as volatile substances have a wide variety of uses in the domestic, school and workplace setting. Some of these preparations are identified in Table 9.1. It is difficult to be certain which ones are used most commonly. The 1994 data for abuse-related deaths [2] showed that gas fuels accounted for nearly two-thirds of all deaths. In previous years the mortality statistics have shown a greater preponderance of aerosols and glues, which seem to be implicated in progressively fewer deaths. It is not clear whether certain volatile substance-based products, and the methods of using them, are intrinsically more likely to cause harm than others or whether a greater awareness of the problem by suppliers and more controls on the sales of glues, in particular, have limited availability.

Note that nitrites are also abused by inhalation but these are discussed in detail in Chapter 17.

As with many forms of drug abuse, VSA can be either a group or an individual activity. The practice can take place in quiet public areas (such as car parks, recreation grounds and woodland) or in the home. The administration methods adopted depend on the inhalant being abused. The abuser needs to obtain a high concentration of volatile substance in the lungs quickly in order to experience the sudden 'rush' of intoxication which is the initial desired effect. To accomplish this, chlorofluorocarbons (CFCs) and butane are sometimes sprayed directly down the throat. This is known to be a very hazardous practice which can cause sudden death (see below).

A far more common procedure is to inhale concentrated fumes from a limited space and to rebreathe this air repeatedly until a 'high' is achieved. Usually this is facilitated by holding a plastic bag containing the inhalant firmly over the mouth and nose and then breathing in and out rapidly several times. This is known as 'huffing'; supermarket carrier bags and crisp packets are commonly used. Other methods have

Table 9.1 Substances which may be abused by inhalation

Substance	Sources
Solvents	
Toluene, xylene, hexane	Many glues (e.g. Bostick, Evostik); paints, paint thinners and paint strippers
1,1,1-Trichloroethane, trichloroethylene	Tippex and other correction fluids (and thinners for them); Zoff (plaster remover); dry cleaning fluids, stain removers, degreasers etc.
Other chlorinated hydrocarbons (eg chloroform, carbon tetra-chloride etc.)	Paints, varnishes, paint strippers, dyestuffs, dry cleaning fluids
Ketones (e.g. acetone)	Nail varnish remover; polystyrene cements
Esters	Marker pens, adhesives
Propellants, gases and fuels	
Propane, butane	Cigarette lighter fuel; bottled camping and stove gases; propellant in aerosols
Chlorofluorocarbons	Propellant in aerosols; active ingredient in PR Spray; fire extinguishers; gaseous general anaesthetics
Dimethyl ether	Aerosol propellant
Nitrous oxide	Entonox; propellant in spray canisters of whipped cream (see Chapter 11)
Fuels	Petrol, paraffin
Nitrites (see Chapter 17)	
Amyl nitrite	Available in sex shops and other outlets
Butyl nitrite	under various brand names

involved placing plastic bags completely over the head or inhaling from underneath bedclothes or similar whole-body covering. Clearly some of these activities carry a risk of death from suffocation.

Many techniques also produce varying degrees of hypoxia, which is known to exacerbate the pro-arrhythmic potential of these agents.

Sometimes abusers breathe fumes directly from the original container; others inhale from hands cupped over the mouth or nose. The inhalant may be applied to clothes (e.g. cuffs and sleeves of jumpers, scarves) or a handkerchief or rag soaked in the solvent can be carried.

PHARMACOKINETICS

Following inhalation, vapours are readily absorbed into the bloodstream and a rapid access to the brain is afforded by the high lipophilicity of the substances involved. The lungs are an important route of excretion subsequent to inhalation. Consequently, being volatile, most solvents and related substances do not cause long-lasting central nervous system (CNS) effects following a single 'sniff' because pulmonary excretion is usually rapid. The actions of butane and CFCs disappear after a few minutes but the effect of toluene can last 30 to 45 minutes following a single 'sniffing' episode.

ADVERSE EFFECTS

The irritant properties of certain solvents such as toluene can produce erythema around the mouth and nose and inflammation of perioral abrasions or spots. Coughing, lacrimation and salivation can also occur as a result of this irritancy. Other undesirable effects from the user's point of view include vomiting, confusion, dizziness and drowsiness. Some abusers become very depressed, aggressive, agitated or frightened.

In 1990, over 4 per cent of all UK deaths in boys aged 10 to 14 years old were caused by inhalant abuse [5]. Deaths are basically the result of one of three consequences: CNS depression, accidents arising as a result of intoxication or sudden death.

All of the inhaled products can cause a CNS derangement which appears superficially similar to drunkenness. Historically, trichloro-ethane, trichloroethylene and chloroform have all been used as general anaesthetics, so the ability of commonly abused inhalants to produce serious CNS depression should not be underestimated. As with all similar drugs, the effects produced in an individual are dose-dependent; greater levels of exposure may result, progressively, in disorientation, ataxia, sedation, unconsciousness and even respiratory depression or coma. In one study of 335 abusers, 3 per cent had been admitted to hospital in a coma and a further 14 per cent had experienced 'blackouts' without hospital admission [6]. There is no evidence that short-term volatile substance abuse causes residual CNS damage or neuropsychological prob-lems [7] but this can occur with chronic exposure [8, 9].

Although the direct CNS effects in isolation are rarely serious, significant repercussions may arise indirectly. Accidental deaths and serious injuries can be sustained by the semiconscious or disorientated abuser, sometimes as a result of hallucinations or illusions; some believe that they are able to fly or swim [10] and falls from heights and drownings do occur. Aspiration of vomit while sedated and suffocation in the large plastic bags used by some teenagers have also been described. In addition, there is a fire risk associated with solvents, fuels and butane propellants because these are highly flammable and many abusers or their associates smoke.

Apart from the direct or indirect CNS effects, the other major cause of mortality is sudden death. Tragically, some of these deaths are in first-time users and, as has already been stated, most of these are young teenagers who would probably only have abused once or twice as an 'experiment'. There are also many fatal cases documented amongst long-term abusers. Most of these deaths are thought to have been due to ventricular fibrillation but this has been difficult to confirm because the majority of sufferers are either found dead or die shortly afterwards. Even when the cause and/or diagnosis has been confirmed at an early stage, resuscitation is often unsuccessful.

Many sudden deaths occur shortly after a bout of 'sniffing' when the abuser is stressed emotionally or physically (particularly by running). It is therefore probable that sympathetic nervous system activity or circulating adrenaline play a role in the aetiology. It seems likely that volatile substances sensitise the myocardium to catecholamines. Animal studies show that both adrenaline [11, 12] and asphyxia [11, 13] increase the arrhythmogenic actions of solvents and that ethanol may further potentiate some of these effects [14].

Animal work also confirms that myocardial sensitivity may persist for hours after inhalant exposure [13]. This may explain why certain documented cases of sudden death seem to occur some time after a sniffing event. The inhalational anaesthetic halothane, itself a CFC, can rarely cause arrhythmias and has even precipitated or exacerbated cardiac problems in those known to have been chronically exposed to solvents [15], providing further evidence that cardiac sensitisation is not always an acute short-lived effect. Interestingly, trichloroethane was used briefly as a general anaesthetic in the 1960s but this practice was discontinued because of a high incidence of ventricular arrhythmias. It is structurally related to halothane.

Another form of sudden death with a cardiac origin is believed to result from vagal inhibition as a reflex response to inhalants being sprayed directly against the back of the throat [16]. Very rapid cooling of the larynx can stimulate the vagus nerve to the extent that the pulse rapidly slows and then the heart stops. This is particularly associated with the butane and CFC propellants.

Although a range of different arrhythmias has been observed in animals exposed to inhalants, ventricular arrhythmias are reported most consistently in humans. Other rare human cardiac effects have included dilated cardiomyopathy [17, 18] and myocardial infarction [19].

Given the many serious risks that the abuser may encounter following inhalation, sniffing by oneself is potentially more hazardous than group activity. Occasionally those presenting with severe arrhythmia are successfully resuscitated [19–21] but this does depend on help being near at hand.

LONG-TERM USE

Generally, chronic abuse may be associated with a decreased ability to concentrate, insomnia and nightmares. Chronic abusers are also more likely to have resorted to theft to keep the habit going. Various medical problems may occur as a result of long-term misuse but there is no consistent pattern to these problems and it is not clear why some abusers suffer and others do not. Adverse effects that have been reported include peripheral and central neurological damage (e.g. peripheral neuropathy, cerebellar damage, encephalopathy), renal failure, hepatoxicity, severe gastrointestinal upset and muscle damage. Some inhalants are more toxic than others; chronic exposure to toluene seems to cause a particularly wide array of adverse effects. Benzene toxicity and lead poisoning have been described in persons regularly exposed to petrol.

Tolerance seems to develop in the chronic user such that much larger amounts of inhalant are required to achieve a 'high'. This tolerance quickly reverses if inhalants are withheld. Dependence of the psychological type can occur after long-term use but physical dependence is less well-known. However, a withdrawal syndrome of irritability, headaches, and delirium tremens-like features has been described in humans [22]. This appears to be rare but usually takes one or two days to develop following abstinence and lasts a further two to five days. Animal work suggests that withdrawal may occur only with certain solvents [1]. On the whole, VSA has a low dependence potential and usually is not associated with chronic daily usage or a compulsion to continue administration.

REDUCING THE PROBLEM

Given the range of potentially abusable substances available, it is virtually impossible to restrict supplies via legislation. The Intoxicating Substances Supply Act of 1985 makes it illegal for any shopkeeper to sell volatile substances with the knowledge that they are likely to be abused but a breach of the law can be difficult to prove. The then

Department of Health and Social Security issued guidelines to shop owners in 1984, suggesting how abusers might be identified and that some products (e.g. adhesives) could be kept behind the counter. It is not illegal to abuse inhalants in public unless the law is broken in other respects (e.g. breach of the peace, criminal damage, trespass).

The retailer needs to appreciate which substances on his/her premises are open to abuse and ensure that all staff understand the nature of the problem. Some products are clearly a greater attraction to abusers than others. For example, of the aerosol products, hairsprays and air fresheners contain a proportionately larger amount of available propellant for abuse than, say, shaving foam or spray paint. These latter products are thus much less likely to be abused. Some products contain virtually pure volatile substances and are particularly open to abuse, e.g. camping stove gas refills, cigarette lighter fuel refills, dry cleaning fluid, PR Spray and correction fluid or paint thinners. Many of these are unusual products for a young teenager to buy and so arouse suspicion. A recent national report in the UK recommended that all potentially abusable household products should be labelled to alert retailers and parents to the potential danger [1]. It is of course difficult to identify a potential abuser; Table 9.2 summarises the key points.

Table 9.2   Pointers to inhalant abuse

- The smell of volatile substances persists on the breath for several hours after inhalation; the smell may also arise from clothes or a cloth about the person
- Frequent purchase of potentially abusable substances by the same individual; groups of teenagers buying inhalants together or suspected shop-lifting of these products
- Signs of intoxication (see text)
- Obvious truancy
- Facial erythema and spots, inflammation or abrasions around the mouth and nose

Additionally for parents

- Finding empty containers of abusable substances or used plastic bags where the teenager has been; signs of glues etc, on skin, clothes or bedclothes
- Regular signs of 'hangover' (e.g. headaches, drowsiness) or of repeated sore throats, coughing or colds
- Sudden changes in mood, lifestyle and appetite, or secrecy concerning absences from home; inability to concentrate

---

Clearly some of these indicators could be confused with the normal process of teenage development.

REFERENCES

1. Advisory Council on the Misuse of Drugs (1995) *Volatile Substance Abuse*, HMSO, London.

2. Taylor, J., Norman, C., Bland, M. and Ramsey, J. (1996) Trends in deaths associated with abuse of volatile substances 1971–1994. Department of Public Health, St George's Hospital Medical School, London.

3. Miller, P.McC. and Plant, M. (1996) Drinking, smoking and illicit drug use among 15 and 16 year olds in the United Kingdom. *Br. Med. J.* **313**: 394–397.

4. Department of Health (1992) *Solvents – a Parent's Guide*, HMSO, London.

5. Anon. (1990) *Drug Misuse in Britain – National Audit of Drug Misuse Statistics*, Institute for the Study of Drug Dependence, London.

6. Watson, J.M. (1986) *Solvent Abuse – Adolescent Epidemic?* Croom Helm, London.

7. Chadwick, O., Anderson, R., Bland, M. and Ramsey, J. (1989) Neuropsychological consequences of volatile substance abuse; a population based study of secondary school pupils. *Br. Med. J.* **298**: 1679–1684.

8. Lolin, Y. (1989) Chronic neurological toxicity associated with exposure to volatile substances. *Hum. Toxicol.* **8**: 293–300.

9. Chadwick, O.F.D. and Anderson, H.R. (1989) Neuropsychological consequences of volatile substance abuse: a review. *Hum. Toxicol.* **8**: 307–312.

10. Evans, A.C. and Raistrick, D. (1987) Phenomenology of intoxication with toluene based adhesives and butane gas. *Br. J. Psychiatr.* **150**: 769–773.

11. Reinhardt, C.F., Azar, A., Maxfield, M.E., Smith, P.E. and Mullin, L.S. (1971) Cardiac arrhythmias and aerosol sniffing. *Arch. Environ. Health,* **22**: 265–279.

12. Clark, D.G. and Tinston, D.J. (1982) Acute inhalation toxicity of some halogenated and non-halogenated hydrocarbons. *Hum. Toxicol.* **1**: 239–247.

13. Taylor, G.J. and Harris, W.S. (1970) Cardiac toxicity of aerosol propellants. *J. Am. Med. Assoc.* **214**: 81–85.

14. White, J. and Carlson, G. (1981) Epinephrine-induced cardiac arrhythmias in rabbits exposed to trichloroethylene: potentiation by ethanol. *Toxicol. Appl. Pharmacol.* **60**: 458–465.

15. McLeod, A.A., Marjot, R., Monaghan, M.J., Hugh-Jones, P. and Jackson, G. (1987) Chronic cardiac toxicity after inhalation of 1,1,1-trichloroethane. *Br. Med. J.* **294**: 727–729.

16. Shepherd, R.T. (1989) Mechanism of sudden death associated with volatile substance abuse. *Hum. Toxicol.* **8**: 287–292.

17. Mee, A.S. and Wright, P.L. (1980) Congested (dilated) cardiomyopathy in association with solvent abuse. *J. R. Soc. Med.* **73**: 671–672.

18. Wiseman, M.N. and Banim, S. (1987) 'Glue sniffer's' heart? *Br. Med. J.* **294**: 739.
19. Cunningham, S.R., Dalzell, G.W.N., McGirr, P. and Khan, M.M. (1987) Myocardial infarction and primary ventricular fibrillation after glue sniffing. *Br. Med. J.* **294**: 739–740.
20. Wodka, R.M. and Jeong, E.W.S. (1989) Cardiac effects of inhaled typewriter correction fluid. *Ann. Intern. Med.* **110**: 91–92.
21. Gunn, J., Wilson, J. and Mackintosh, A.F. (1989) Butane sniffing causing ventricular fibrillation. *Lancet*, **333**: 617.
22. Merry, J. and Zachariadis, N. (1962) Addiction to glue sniffing. *Br. Med. J.* **2**: 1448.

FURTHER READING

1. Volatile substance abuse. *Hum. Toxicol.* 1989; **8(4)**: complete issue pp. 255–334.
2. Ives, R. (1990) Helping the sniffers. *Druglink*, **5**: pp.10–13.
3. Sharp, C.W., Beauvais, F. and Spence, R. (eds) (1992) Inhalant abuse: a volatile research agenda, *NIDA Res. Monogr.* **129**.

10

Performance enhancing drugs

Man is a gaming animal. He must always be trying to get the better in something or other.
Charles Lamb (1775–1834), 'Essays of Elia'.

A huge range of drugs have been used to enhance athletic and gymnastic performance, to increase strength, assist in training, boost stamina or promote a muscular physique. Stimulant drugs such as amphetamines, cocaine, over-the-counter sympathomimetics and caffeine have been used widely to enhance performance in endurance sports and to increase stamina during training but these are the subject of other chapters in this book. Similarly, cannabis has been used to promote calmness and relaxation for events where this is desirable. The remaining substances discussed below range from simple chemical elements to complex naturally occurring proteins. Many of the preparations used are nutritional supplements and a detailed discussion of these is beyond the scope of this book. However, some individual nutrients are highlighted.

ANABOLIC STEROIDS

Anabolic steroids are the classic performance enhancing drugs; associated with Soviet Block athletes in the Cold War, cheating at the Olympics and a range of unpleasant side effects. So much so that the generic term 'steroid', which incorporates a wide range of drugs used therapeutically from vitamin D to oral contraceptives, has become synonymous with anabolic steroid in the minds of many members of the public.

Abuse of anabolic steroids has become increasingly prevalent in the West during the past decade. In the USA, both the possession and supply of these drugs was declared illegal in 1990. In the UK the situation is more complex. It is not illegal to import anabolic steroids from outside the UK as long as these are for personal use. Consequently, possession of anabolic steroids in the form of a medicinal product is also not illegal. However, possession of anabolic steroids in the form of raw materials (i.e. unformulated) was made a criminal act under new legislation in September 1996. An offence is also committed if anabolic steroids are supplied in any form to another private individual within the UK without a prescription.

Effects sought

Anabolic steroids are taken to increase skeletal muscle mass, and physical strength. They also increase stamina, decrease fatigue and may even cause a mild euphoria. Such effects are particularly important because they enable users to train longer and harder. They also increase the risk of muscle and other body damage which is detrimental to the desired effects. The effectiveness of anabolic steroids in increasing the physical strength of an individual is open to doubt. Intensively trained athletes who take them may benefit if a vigorous training schedule is maintained in association with a high protein, high calorie diet [1] but otherwise an improvement in strength may not occur.

Although anabolic steroids were initially abused mainly by international athletes, there has been a dramatic increase in the variety of users in the past decade. Bodybuilders, aspiring athletes and 'keep-fit' fanatics are some of the more obvious groups involved. However, anabolic steroids are increasingly taken by those who desire a more muscular physique for cosmetic purposes or who require increased aggression. Most of these also engage in weight training. In one study of attenders at gymnasia in Swansea, nearly 40 per cent of those questioned had taken anabolic steroids [2]. A survey of 633 students attending a Scottish technical college in 1993 revealed an incidence of anabolic steroid use of 2.8 per cent [3]. A larger UK study of 1659 gym participants from across the country was also described in 1993; it revealed a 7.7 per cent incidence of anabolic steroid use amongst men and women but the incidence was 9.1 per cent amongst men alone [4]. Use amongst schoolchildren is also increasing. An investigation into the drug-taking habits of 7722 UK pupils aged 15 and 16 years old in 1996 found that 1 per cent girls and 2.2 per cent boys had used steroids on at least one occasion [5]. A summary of surveys of secondary schoolchildren in the USA showed that between 1.4 per cent and 10.9 per cent of them had used anabolic steroids [6]. In all studies in the US and UK a significantly greater proportion of users are male.

Administration

The drugs used are basically analogues of testosterone and examples are listed in Table 10.1. Administration is via the oral or intramuscular route; the latter is more popular but frequently both routes are used simultaneously. Testosterone cannot be given orally because the high rate of first-pass metabolism in the liver results in inadequate plasma concentrations; the intramuscular route is therefore mandatory. Anabolic steroid injections are formulated in oil which allows a sustained release of drug from the intramuscular site over a period of weeks or days. A certain amount of discomfort or pain after injection is common, especially if the volume of a single injection exceeds 4 ml.

The doses used are usually considerably in excess of those used therapeutically – typically 10 to 100 times greater – and it is common for more than one anabolic steroid to be used at the same time. This practice is referred to as 'stacking'. Mixing different anabolic steroids in the same syringe is called 'blending'. Steroids are often taken intensively for a duration of 6 to 12 weeks and the course is then repeated after a suitable interval. This is termed 'cycling'. Commonly the dose of each steroid is started at a low level, built up to a maximum halfway through the course and then tapered off towards the end, a technique known as 'pyramiding'. If a particular drug appears to become ineffective after a period of time ('plateauing') then users usually switch to another.

Adverse effects

Testosterone, the hormone on which other anabolic steroids are based, has both androgenic and anabolic actions. None of the synthetic derivatives is devoid of androgenic effects, and these are responsible for a

Table 10.1 Some of the more common anabolic steroid preparations

Generic name	Proprietary name
Drostanolone	Masteril, Drolban
Methandienone	Danabol
Methenolone	Primobolan
Nandrolone	Durabolin, Deca-durabolin
Oxandrolone	Anavar
Oxymetholone	Anapolon
Stanozolol	Stromba
Testosterone	Sustanon

high proportion of the side effects seen in the abuser. It has not proved possible to synthesise an anabolic steroid which is devoid of these masculinising qualities. Almost all of the side effects of anabolic steroids are dose-dependent and are more likely when prolonged administration occurs.

In men, the large doses of anabolic steroids used commonly depress the pituitary–testicular axis giving rise to testicular atrophy and oligospermia or azoospermia. Any sperm which are produced are more likely to be abnormal. The amount of semen produced is also less. Increased or decreased libido may occur. Impotence is quite common but priapism is rare and tends to be associated with very high doses. Usually all these effects are reversible.

Anabolic steroids can be metabolised to female sex hormones by the liver which can produce feminising effects in men in the presence of suppressed testosterone production [7]. For example, gynaecomastia is a recognised effect and often the breasts are painful or tender. 'Hot flushing' is another well-known problem.

The prostate gland tends to enlarge and existing prostate problems are made worse. This may result in impaired micturition.

In women, anabolic steroids tend to cause irregular, smaller, infrequent menstruations or amenorrhoea, and reduced fertility. Virilisation may occur with increased growth of hair on the body and face, deepening of the voice, enlargement of the clitoris, increased libido and reduced breast size. Anabolic steroids may make it impossible to breast feed. Unfortunately, most of these effects are permanent and do not improve when anabolic steroids are stopped.

Anabolic steroids cause sodium (fluid) retention. This can worsen hypertension and could theoretically exacerbate heart/kidney disorders, epilepsy, migraine or diabetes. Long-term use seems to increase the risk of thrombosis [8], myocardial infarction [9], pulmonary embolus [10], stroke [11], ischaemic heart disease and hypertension. Anabolic steroids can increase the blood concentrations of low-density lipoprotein cholesterol and decrease beneficial high-density lipoprotein levels [12].

Cancer caused by anabolic steroids is rare. However, abuse has been recognised as a rare cause of cancer of the liver [13–15] and other cancers have been reported including those of the prostate [16] and kidney [17]. Brygden et al. [17] suggest that these may arise due to the relatively higher levels of tumorigenic circulating oestrogen and the hypertrophic effects of synthetic androgens.

Relatives and friends of an anabolic steroid user commonly confide that an individual's personality has changed since commencing abuse. As a result of these observations, the effects of anabolic steroids on the mind have been investigated in some detail [18–21]. Initially use of anabolic steroids may produce stimulatory effects such as increased confidence, decreased fatigue, heightened motivation, agitation, irritability and insomnia. This may progress so that users become argumentative, impetuous, moody, suspicious and aggressive. Eventually dangerous, violent and antisocial behaviour may occur. Not uncommonly, violent periodic outbursts of temper are reported ('roid rages') particularly when large doses are taken for a long time.

Anabolic steroid use may also cause frank psychiatric illness such as depression, severe paranoia and psychosis. A recent review highlighted that weight-training itself may cause some personality and mood changes, and increased assertiveness [22]. This possibility is not always taken into consideration in studies of the effects of anabolic steroids on personality.

It is not clear whether anabolic steroids can cause physical dependence; some case reports suggest that this might occur in certain individuals. However, these drugs do *not* cause addisonian-like withdrawal reactions akin to those produced by glucocorticosteroids so abrupt cessation is acceptable.

Injecting any drug carries the risk of injection site infection as well as systemic infection such as septicaemia. In one study [2], 13 per cent of users acknowledged that they had shared injecting equipment or loaned it to someone else, thus increasing the risk of infections such as AIDS and hepatitis. Another study showed an incidence of 16 per cent [23]. AIDS cases in injecting steroid abusers have been reported [24, 25]. Concern has been expressed that this population is not as well-informed as other parenteral drug abusers concerning the risks of HIV transmission via shared needles. The chance of sharing may be raised because the larger bore needles needed for intramuscular injection of these viscous solutions may not be as easily available as the narrower gauge intravenous varieties.

A link between regular anabolic steroid use and immunosuppression has not been proven but has been suggested by some authors. For example, two cases of infections characteristic of immunosuppression in otherwise healthy anabolic steroid users led to speculation that the link might go unnoticed because of failure to identify anabolic steroid use. One case involved sight-threatening *Candida albicans* endophthalmitis [26] and the other severe chickenpox pneumonitis [27]. A survey of 70 anabolic steroid users in North Wales discovered that 54 per cent of those questioned reported 'frequent colds' as a side effect [23].

Cholestatic jaundice with concomitant abnormal liver function tests can be caused by anabolic steroids [13, 28] because they have a dose-dependent ability to inhibit bile production. The condition appears to be reversible in almost all cases.

Acne and alopecia are common side effects in both sexes. Abusers may take antibiotics or topical retinoids to counteract drug-induced acne. Reduced growth and short stature is likely in children and young teenagers due to premature closure of the epiphyses. At all ages, anabolic steroids may increase the risk of tendon damage on exercise. Over-exercise can trigger rhabdomyolysis and its sequelae [29].

Accessory drugs associated with anabolic steroid use

A whole range of other drugs may be abused by athletes to counteract the side effects of anabolic steroids or to augment their effects. Some common examples are highlighted below.

Diuretics

Diuretics counteract the fluid retention caused by anabolic steroids and may sharpen the definition of skeletal muscle contours.

Tamoxifen

This drug helps to reduce the gynaecomastia which may develop as a side effect of anabolic steroid use. Gynaecomastia is not only unsightly but can also be painful.

Human chorionic gonadotrophin

Human chorionic gonadotrophin (HCG) stimulates the Leydig cells of the testis to increase secretion of testosterone thus theoretically minimising the adverse effects of a depressed pituitary–testicular axis. It is given intramuscularly, usually in association with anabolic steroids, but at least two cases are known in which HCG was taken alone with purportedly the desired anabolic effects.

Growth hormone (somatropin)

There is little evidence that growth hormone has any beneficial effects on muscle mass or athletic performance. Supplies from illicit sources may be of poor quality and very expensive; this also applies to HCG. Concern has been expressed in the past that illicit growth hormone with a cadaveric source has increased the risk of users developing

Creutzfeldt–Jakob disease [29, 30]. Prolonged excessive use of growth hormone can cause adverse reactions reminiscent of acromegaly.

Thyroxine

Thyroxine increases the rate of metabolism, which might theoretically increase the ability of anabolic steroids to boost physical strength. Thyroxine also encourages rapid utilisation of a high calorie diet.

CLENBUTEROL

This drug is a long-acting beta-2 adrenoceptor agonist which is used medicinally in some European countries as an oral bronchodilator. Clenbuterol is not licensed as a medicine for human use in the UK or USA. It is abused by bodybuilders and athletes because it supposedly has anabolic-like effects, although some scientists refer to clenbuterol as a 'repartitioning' agent because the mode of action is not the same as that of anabolic steroids.

In several species of animal, clenbuterol increases the bulk of certain groups of skeletal muscles and reduces the amount of subcutaneous fat [31, 32]. The doses required for this effect are greater than those needed for bronchodilation. These experiments in animals have been extrapolated to humans by proponents of the use of clenbuterol. However, it is often the case that drugs which produce one effect in animals do not produce the same effect in humans and the actions of clenbuterol have not been studied in humans or any closely related species such as primates. Another limitation of the laboratory work available is that, unlike the human athletes who take it, the animal species involved were not engaged in regular heavy exercise and were studied under controlled conditions. Animal work also shows that skeletal muscles are affected unequally and the importance of this observation to the hopeful athlete or bodybuilder is not clear.

The typical dose taken for an anabolic effect in man is 60 to 120 micrograms daily, usually in the form of 20 microgram tablets. Interestingly, clenbuterol has been reported as an adulterant of anabolic steroid injections in sufficient quantities (2 mg) to cause toxicity after injection [33].

The mechanism of action is not clearly understood but the drug may produce an initial increase in the rate of skeletal muscle protein synthesis which is then subsequently accompanied by a drug-induced decrease in the rate of protein breakdown [34]. This has led to interest in the therapeutic potential of clenbuterol for treating conditions where muscle wastage can occur due to sepsis, immobility or cachexia.

GAMMA HYDROXYBUTYRATE [35–37]

This drug is also known as 4-hydroxybutyrate, hydroxybutyric acid, sodium oxybate, GHB, GBH or liquid X. It is usually supplied as a white powder, sometimes as capsules or occasionally tablets. It is not subject to the Misuse of Drugs Act in the UK but it is a prescription-only drug so unauthorised synthesis or supply without a prescription is illegal. As is the case with anabolic steroids, GHB can be lawfully imported into the country for personal use.

GHB is actually a product of normal human metabolism that is known to increase dopamine concentrations in the brain and to interact with endogenous central nervous system opioids. It is a catabolite of the inhibitory neurotransmitter GABA and is found at 1000-fold lower concentrations than GABA itself. It may be a neurotransmitter in its own right as transport mechanisms and binding sites have been identified in the brain [38]. GHB has been used medicinally as an adjunct to anaesthesia, to alleviate the symptoms of narcolepsy, to treat alcoholism and heroin addiction, and to ameliorate the effects of cerebral ischaemia in patients with head injuries.

GHB is taken orally, usually dissolved in water, although occasional reports of injection are described. Doses range from 2 g to over 30 g. It is claimed to be an alternative to anabolic steroids which purportedly increases muscle bulk and reduces body fat by stimulating the secretion of growth hormone. In addition GHB has been abused because it has sedative properties and it can produce a prolonged euphoria which may last in excess of 24 hours. The sedative effects, if undesirable, can be counteracted by administration with a stimulant such as amphetamine. Psychoactive effects are generally potentiated when taken with other psychotropic substances but begin about 15 to 60 minutes after ingestion.

Table 10.2 Adverse effects of GHB

- Drowsiness, hypnagogic states, confusion, agitation, amnesia, unconsciousness, respiratory depression, coma
- Nausea, vomiting, diarrhoea
- Ataxia, hypotonia, myoclonic seizure-like episodes, tremors, headache, possibly extrapyramidal symptoms
- Vertigo, dizziness
- Bradycardia, hypotension
- Hypothermia
- Metabolic acidosis, hypernatraemia, hyperglycaemia

GHB is metabolised to carbon dioxide and water alone; there are no active metabolites. The human elimination half-life has been measured as about 20 to 30 minutes for small doses [39, 40] but it has been suggested that the elimination pathway is saturable and that at high doses the half-life would effectively be increased as a result.

Side effects are summarised in Table 10.2. GHB was reported to cause a withdrawal reaction in one patient [41]. A 30 year old woman who had taken 25 g daily in five divided doses for two years decreased the dose to 10 g per day before stopping completely. Twelve hours after the last dose she experienced tremor, anxiety and insomnia which persisted for 12 days after cessation, but then resolved. Subsequent to this report several other cases of a withdrawal reaction have been described [47].

NATURAL PRODUCTS AND NUTRITIONAL SUPPLEMENTS

A survey of advertisements for nutritional supplements in UK body-building magazines in 1994 identified 145 different products. Of these, 53 per cent contained vitamins and/or metal cations and 19 per cent disclosed no ingredients at all. The most popular claim, made by one-third of advertisements, was that of enhanced performance. Other common claims were: assisting muscle gain, promoting weight reduction and a 'general supplement' [42]. The author of the report highlighted that, in the UK, as long as no medicinal claims are made, the manufacturers of nutritional products can make any claims they wish about the benefits of using their preparations. No scientific evidence is necessary to back up such claims.

Many preparations are simply mixtures of protein, amino acids, carbohydrate, fats, minerals and/or vitamins in varying proportion. Others contain more specific, unusual, or exotic ingredients. Whatever the formulation, any claims of efficacy that are made are often unreasonable extrapolations from animal studies or from unrepresentative or limited human exposure. Table 10.3 lists some of the ingredients which have been identified in such products [42–45]. Vitamins are not included in this table although most of them can be found in various guises in such products. Vitamins C, B_{12} and E are probably the most popular. Although certain ingredients have been studied in some detail, none of them has been tested adequately enough in humans to fully support the claims made for them.

In summary, these products are marketed with no, or very little, evidence of efficacy or safety. Often details of dosage or contraindications are lacking. Without detailed study in humans such products

Table 10.3 Ingredients found in natural or nutritional products used by athletes and bodybuilders

Ingredient	Claimed beneficial effects
Animal organs	Extracts of these are found in some preparations, with a variety of claims; liver, testes, pituitary and pancreas are examples
Arginine	Amino acid claimed to increase release of growth hormone
Bee pollen	Increased speed of recovery after exercise
Boron	Augments action of testosterone
L-Carnitine	Promotes loss of body fat; decreased lactic acid production; sparing of muscle glycogen
Choline	Promotes loss of body fat
Chromium	Anabolic compound, usually supplied as picolinate salt
Co-Enzyme Q10	Increased performance, increased oxidative metabolism
Diosgenin	Substitute for steroids, due to similar structure
Ethoxyquin	Antioxidant
Ferulic acid	Anabolic effect
Gamma Oryzanol	Anabolic effect
Ginseng	Improved and/or prolonged performance in endurance events
Inosine	Energy enhancer; increased oxygen release to muscle
Medium chain triglycerides	Increased energy and reduced body fat
Octacosanol	Ergogenic effects
Ornithine	As for arginine
Phosphate	Enhanced energy utilisation
Silymarin	Liver protection
Smilax spp.	Natural source of testosterone or testosterone enhancer
Yohimbine	Natural source of testosterone or testosterone enhancer

should be viewed at best as a waste of money and no substitute for a professionally organised and supervised training programme.

PRESCRIPTION MEDICINES

Anabolic steroids and the accessory drugs discussed above, together with clenbuterol and gamma hydroxybutyrate, are all prescription medicines in the UK. Consequently, supply by any person in the UK to another individual in the UK is illegal without a prescription. This also applies to the drugs discussed below.

Beta blockers

These can decrease tremor and pulse in sports where intense concentration and a steady hand are a necessity, e.g. archery, shooting, darts, snooker.

Diltiazem

Diltiazem is not a drug that would be expected to enhance performance in a healthy adult. However, a report in 1993 described a man who took 480 mg of diltiazem per day and developed severe abdominal cramps as a result [46]. He revealed that the drug was widely abused amongst bodybuilders and rugby players locally to augment training but the exact benefits that he anticipated from the drug were not made clear.

Diuretics

These may be taken to promote a rapid short-lasting weight loss prior to 'weighing in' before competitions where exceeding a maximum weight may result in disqualification.

Erythropoietin

There is a belief among certain elements of the sporting community that increasing plasma haemoglobin, and thence the oxygen carrying capacity of the blood, is beneficial to muscular function during sustained physical exercise. Blood transfusions are given to achieve this but erythropoietin is also used because it increases the rate of production of red blood cells. However, there are dangers involved in this practice. Strenuous exercise is known to promote haemoconcentration due to loss of fluid and this in turn results in increased blood viscosity. Elevating the red blood cell concentration has a similar effect on viscosity so erythropoietin administration may increase the risk of thrombosis during exercise.

Drugs that stimulate release of growth hormone

Clonidine, levodopa and vasopressin can all stimulate growth hormone production and each one has been abused for this effect.

REFERENCES

1. Kibble, M.W. and Ross, M.B. (1987) Adverse effects of anabolic steroids in athletes. *Clin. Pharm.* **6**: 686–692.
2. Perry, H.M., Wright, D. and Littlepage, N.C. (1992) Dying to be big: a review of anabolic steroid use. *Br. J. Sports Med.* **26**: 259–261.
3. Williamson, D.J. (1993) Misuse of anabolic drugs (letter). *Br. Med. J.* **306**: 61.
4. Korkia, P. and Stimson, G.V. (1993) *Anabolic Steroid Use in Great Britain: an Exploratory Investigation*, HMSO, London.
5. Miller, P.McC. and Plant, M. (1996) Drinking, smoking, and illicit drug use among 15 and 16 year olds in the United Kingdom. *Br. Med. J.* **313**: 394–397.
6. Yesalis, C.E. and Bahrke, M.S. (1995) Anabolic-androgenic steroids. *Sports Med.* **19**: 326–340.
7. Knuth, U.A., Maniera, H. and Nieschlag, E. (1989) Anabolic steroids and semen parameters in bodybuilders. *Fertil. Steril.* **52**: 1041–1047.
8. Ferenchick, G.S. (1991) Are androgenic steroids thrombogenic? *N. Engl. J. Med.* **322**: 476.
9. Kennedy, M.C. and Lawrence, C. (1993) Anabolic steroid abuse and cardiac death. *Med. J. Aust.* **158**: 346–348.
10. Robinson, R.J. and White, S. (1993) Misuse of anabolic drugs (letter). *Br. Med. J.* **306**: 61.
11. Ferenchick, G.S. (1991) Drug abuse and stroke (letter). *Ann. Intern. Med.* **114**: 431.
12. Glazer, G. (1991) Atherogenic effects of anabolic steroids on serum lipid levels. *Arch. Intern . Med.* **151**: 1923–1933.
13. Farrell, G.C. (1994) *Drug-induced Liver Disease*, Churchill Livingstone, London, pp. 177, 334.
14. Overly, W.L., Dankoff, J.A., Wang, B.K. and Singh, U.D. (1984) Androgens and hepatocellular carcinoma in an athlete (letter). *Ann. Intern. Med.* **100**: 158–159.
15. Goldman, B. (1985) Liver carcinoma in an athlete taking anabolic steroids (letter). *J. Am. Osteopath. Assoc.* **85**: 56.
16. Roberts, J.T. and Essenhigh, D.M. (1986) Letter. *Lancet,* **2**: 742.
17. Brygden, A.A.G., Rothwell, P.J.N. and O'Reilly, P.H. (1995) Anabolic steroid abuse and renal-cell carcinoma (letter). *Lancet,* **346**: 1307–1308.
18. Smith, D.A. and Perry, P.J. (1992) The efficacy of ergogenic agents in athletic competition. Part I: Androgenic-anabolic steroids. *Ann. Pharmacother.* **26**: 520–528.
19. Parrott, A.C., Choi, P.Y.L. and Davies, M. (1994) Anabolic steroid use by amateur athletes: effects upon psychological mood state. *J. Sports Med. Phys. Fit.* **34**: 292–298.
20. Cooper, C.J., Noakes, T.D., Dunne, T., Lambert, M.I. and Rochford, K. (1996) A high prevalence of abnormal personality traits in chronic users of anabolic-androgenic steroids. *Br. J. Sports Med.* **30**: 246–250.

21. Corrigan, B. (1996) Anabolic steroids and the mind. *Med. J. Aust.* **165**: 222–226.

22. Bahrke, M.S. and Yesalis, C.E. (1994) Weight training – a potential confounding factor in examining the psychological and behavioural effects of anabolic-androgenic steroids. *Sports Med.* **18**: 309–318.

23. Burton, C. (1996) Anabolic steroid use among the gym population in Clwyd. *Pharm. J.* **256**: 557–559.

24. Scott, M.J. and Scott, M.J. (Jr) (1989) HIV infection associated with injections of anabolic steroids. *J. Am. Med. Assoc.* **262**: 207–208.

25. Sklarek, H.M., Mantovani, R.P., Erens, E., Heisler, D., Neiderman, M.S. and Fein, A.M. (1984) AIDS in a bodybuilder using anabolic steroids. *N. Engl. J. Med.* **311**: 1701.

26. Widder, R.A., Bartz-Schmidt, K.U., Geter, H. *et al.* (1995) *Candida albicans* endophthalmitis after anabolic steroid abuse (letter). *Lancet*, **345**: 330–331.

27. Johnson, A.S., Jones, M., Morgan-Capner, P. *et al.* (1995) Severe chickenpox in anabolic steroid user (letter). *Lancet*, **345**: 1447–1448.

28. Lowdell, C.P. and Murray-Lyon, I.M. (1985) Reversal of liver damage due to long term methyltestosterone and safety of non-17 alpha-alkylated androgens. *Br. Med. J.* **291**: 637.

29. Shotliff, K. and Asante, M. (1993) Misuse of anabolic drugs (letter). *Br. Med. J.* **306**: 61–62.

30. Deyssig, R. and Frisch, H. (1993) Self-administration of cadaveric growth hormone in power athletes (letter). *Lancet*, **341**:768–769.

31. Prather, I.D., Brown, D.E., North, P. and Wilson, J.R. (1995) Clenbuterol: A substitute for anabolic steroids? *Med. Sci. Sports Exercise*, **27**: 1118–1121.

32. Spann, C. and Winter, M.E. (1995) Effect of clenbuterol on athletic performance. *Ann. Pharmacother.* **29**: 75–77.

33. Lenehan, P. (1996) Information letter from the Drugs and Sport Information Service, *Warning: Counterfeit Anabolic Steroid Health Risk – Anabol*, Room 159, 9 Slater Street, Liverpool L15 1HB, UK.

34. Anon. (1992) Muscling in on clenbuterol. *Lancet*, **340**: 403.

35. Dyer, J.E., Kreutzer, R., Quatrone, A. *et al.* (1991) Multistate outbreak of poisonings associated with illicit use of gamma hydroxybutyrate. *J. Am. Med. Assoc.* **265**: 447–448.

36. Anon. (1991) From the Food and Drug Administration: Warning about GHB. *J. Am. Med. Assoc.* **265**: 1802.

37. Anon. (1995) *Gamma Hydroxybutyric Acid (GHB) Intoxication: Clinical Features and Management*, National Poisons Information Service, London, pp. 1–3.

38. Cash, C.D. (1994) Gammahydroxybutyrate. An overview of the pros and cons for it being a neurotransmitter and/or a useful therapeutic agent. *Neurosci. Biobehav. Rev.* **18**: 291–304.

39. Ferrara, S.D., Zotti, S., Tedeschi, L. *et al.* (1992) Pharmacokinetics of gamma-hydroxybutyric acid in alcohol dependent patients after single and repeated oral doses. *Br. J. Clin. Pharmacol.* **34**: 231–235.

40. Palatini, P., Tedeschi, L., Frison, G. *et al.* (1993) Dose-dependent absorption and elimination of gamma-hydroxybutyric acid in healthy volunteers. *Eur. J. Clin. Pharmacol.* **45**: 353–356.

41. Galloway, G.P., Frederick, S.L. and Staggers (Jr), F. (1994) Physical dependence on sodium oxybate (letter). *Lancet*, **343**: 57.

42. Timmins, A.J. (1994) Survey of advertisements for nutritional supplements in bodybuilding magazines. *Pharm. J.* **253**: 894–895.

43. Beltz, S.D. and Doering, P.L. (1993) Efficacy of nutritional supplements used by athletes. *Clin. Pharm.* **12**: 900–908.

44. Grunewald, K.K. and Bailey, R.S. (1993) Commercially marketed supplements for bodybuilding athletes. *Sports Med.* **15**: 90–103.

45. Barron, R.L. and Vanscoy, G.J. (1993) Natural products and the athlete: facts and folklore. *Ann. Pharmacother.* **27**: 607–615.

46. Richards, H., Grocutt, M. and McCabe, M. (1993) Use of diltiazem in sport (letter). *Br. Med. J.* **307**: 940.

47 Galloway, G.P., Frederick, S.L., Staggers (Jr), F.E. *et al.* (1997) Gamma hydroxybutyrate: an emerging drug of abuse that causes physical dependence. *Addiction* **92**: 89–96.

11

Prescription drugs

The medicine increases the disease.
Virgil (70–19BC), 'The Aeneid'.

This chapter highlights the important areas of abuse of prescription drugs. Opioids, cocaine, dexamphetamine, anabolic steroids and many of their derivatives are prescription medicines in the UK but these have been the subject of earlier chapters. Similarly, some 'smart drugs' and certain preparations used in association with anabolic steroids are also prescription drugs and are discussed elsewhere in this book.

ANAESTHETICS

Many gaseous anaesthetics have been subject to abuse but in practice these all have a low abuse potential because although they may produce pleasurable effects they are not easily available and are inconvenient to use, even for healthcare professionals with access to them. The exception is ketamine abuse which is a well-described problem at street level.

Nitrous oxide

Nitrous oxide gas is not a prescription medicine in the UK but is included in this chapter for ease of reference. It is used therapeutically to induce anaesthesia and also as an analgesic. In this setting it is usually mixed with oxygen and is available commercially as Entonox in characteristic blue and white cylinders (Figure 11.1). Abuse is most likely to involve healthcare personnel who use nitrous oxide in the workplace, e.g. dentists, anaesthetists and theatre staff. However, the gas is also the propellant used in many canisters of pressurised whipped cream. The

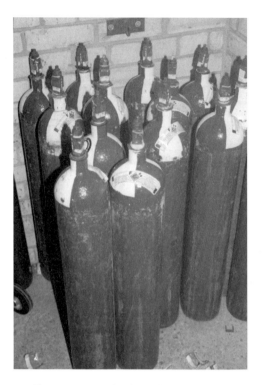

Figure 11.1 Cylinders of Entonox gas.

experienced abuser is able to release the gas into containers, allowing subsequent gas inhalation with minimum cream contamination. Inhalation
is usually via a plastic bag, balloon or similar device. Healthcare staff may,
of course, use anaesthetic administration equipment. In 1979, a US survey of 524 medical and dental students showed that 16 per cent of those
questioned had abused nitrous oxide on at least one occasion [1].

Acute exposure to nitrous oxide can produce a short-lasting pleasurable intoxication: euphoria, relaxation, feelings of detachment and
merriment (hence the alternative name of 'laughing gas'). The mechanism behind these central nervous system (CNS) effects is not fully
understood but research suggests that it may, to a greater or lesser extent,
be the result of an agonist action at central opioid receptors. This could
be a direct action on opioid receptors, augmentation of the effects of
endogenous opioids or stimulation of their release [2, 3].

The cognitive impairment produced usually lasts only a few minutes
because the gas is rapidly excreted via the lungs. Inhalation of the pure
gas without oxygen (i.e. non-Entonox sources) can cause acute hypoxia
either via oxygen insufficiency during inhalation or by nitrous oxide

displacement of oxygen from alveoli during the excretion of the gas from the body. This latter mechanism – diffusion hypoxia – can be fatal.

As with volatile substance abuse, the results of intoxication are potentially more dangerous than the direct effect of the gas itself because accidents can occur in the disorientated abuser. Nitrous oxide can sometimes cause nausea or vomiting; consequently there is a small risk of aspiration of vomit. Unlike many chemicals subject to volatile substance abuse, nitrous oxide is not flammable and it also does not itself seem to cause 'sudden death' in the same manner as volatile substances (see Chapter 9). However, some fresh cream aerosol canisters with a nitrous oxide propellant may contain other propellants, such as chlorofluorocarbons, and nitrous oxide itself may produce degrees of hypoxia, as mentioned above. These two factors theoretically increase the risk of arrhythmia. In a review of 11 fatal cases of abuse the cause of death, when it could be determined, was attributed to asphyxiation, fatal accident or aspiration of vomit [4]. Fainting [1], pneumomediastinum [5] and frostbite [6] have also been reported as acute effects.

Repeated abuse has been associated with the development of a range of severe neurological disorders (mostly myeloneuropathies and neuropathies) and bone marrow depression. These adverse effects are believed to be caused by nitrous oxide accelerating vitamin B_{12} breakdown. Neurological damage is usually at least partly reversible but recovery is often slow and incomplete [7–10]. Bone marrow depression is more quickly and completely reversible but has proved a serious complication in acutely ill patients administered long-term, high-dose nitrous oxide for therapeutic reasons [9, 11]. Cases of psychosis have been attributed to long-term use of the gas [12–14]. Physical dependence may occur following chronic regular use, a delirium-like withdrawal state having been described in one patient [13] but this is probably extremely rare.

Ketamine

Therapeutically, ketamine is used by the intravenous or intramuscular routes to induce or maintain anaesthesia. It has been known for many years that patients in recovery following ketamine anaesthesia may experience psychotomimetic reactions. These 'emergence' phenomena commonly include feelings of mind–body dissociation (so-called 'out-of-the-body experiences'), sensations of floating, severe disorientation, vivid dreams and even delirium. Any of these effects may be subjectively pleasant or unpleasant.

Unlike the other anaesthetic agents described here, illicit supplies of ketamine are available on the street. Commercially ketamine is only available in a parenteral formulation, and although it has been abused by injection, it seems to be more popular as an oral intoxicant. Eastman *et al.* reported in 1992 that an oral formulation might be prepared by evaporation of water from the injection solution, followed by packing into capsules [15]. The drug can also be inhaled into the nose as a dry powder ('snorting'). Street names for ketamine include 'K', 'vitamin K', 'super K', 'special K' and 'kit-kat'. The drug is sometimes detected as an adulterant in other illicit drugs, especially ecstasy, but it is used quite widely in its own right. The prevalence of abuse in Sweden has been such that legislation has been proposed to curtail usage [16].

Although an anaesthetic agent, ketamine only causes respiratory depression after very high doses. The main danger from abuse arises from the peculiarly altered states of consciousness that it can produce. Individuals may become so divorced from reality that the surrounding environment is perceived completely differently by the abuser. He or she may genuinely experience a 'different world'. This is called dissociation. In this respect, ketamine intoxication has some similarities to the effects of phencyclidine to which it is structurally related (see Chapter 8). This, coupled with delusions of paralysis or difficulty in moving and the analgesic effects of ketamine, could obviously result in serious accidents, depending on the location of the abuser. Ketamine has the potential to cause memory impairment, persistent repetitive movements (stereotypies) and can also give rise to 'flashbacks' [17].

Other anaesthetics

Historically, anaesthetic ether was subject to abuse in the same way as most volatile liquids have been. Ether is now never used as an anaesthetic in the West and supplies are difficult for the potential user to obtain. Some of the simple chlorinated alkanes (e.g. 1,1,1-trichloroethane) abused as solvents today have also been employed as anaesthetics in the past. There are occasional reports of abuse of more modern gaseous anaesthetics, e.g. enflurane [18, 19], cyclopropane [20], halothane [21] and fluothane [22]. In each case abuse of these substances was reported in the medical literature because the abuser died as a result. Inhalational anaesthetics such as these are similar to many of the chemicals subject to volatile substance abuse – a well-known cause of sudden death (see Chapter 9). Halothane abuse has been cited as a cause of hepatitis, a rare idiosyncratic side-effect when the drug is used an anaesthetic [23]. Ethyl chloride has also been abused by inhalation [24]; this product is sometimes used as a topical anaesthetic.

ANTIDEPRESSANTS

All antidepressants serve to increase the concentration of certain neurotransmitters in the brain: principally dopamine, noradrenaline and serotonin. Illicit drugs such as cocaine and amphetamines also boost the concentrations of these substances in the CNS and this property is known to be important for producing psychotropic effects. It is not surprising therefore that antidepressants themselves have been the subject of abuse. However, the total number of cases reported over the past 30 years is very small. Consequently, it has been argued that patients should not be informed of the abuse potential because the benefits of warning about the tiny risk of abuse are outweighed by the risk of causing non-compliance with a medication that can be life-saving (by preventing suicide) [25]. However, other authors feel that the patient should be warned in a non-alarmist way [26].

Monoamine oxidase inhibitors

Tranylcypromine is the monoamine oxidase inhibitor (MAOI) that has been abused most commonly. It has an amphetamine-like structure and has been abused for its stimulant-like effects. Most reported cases have involved patients with a history of depression who discovered that taking 100 to 300 mg of tranylcypromine per day resolved depression and produced a sense of well-being [26–31]. Abuse of phenelzine has also been reported at a dosage of 90 to 150 mg per day [31]. As with tranylcypromine, patients reported stimulant effects from these high doses. Some abusers have reported withdrawal reactions upon discontinuation.

Moclobemide, a selective inhibitor of CNS monoamine oxidase A, has abused to produce euphoria in combination with citalopram or clomipramine [32]. The authors of the report do not provide details of the doses used but do reveal that five individuals involved in this practice died from the serotonin syndrome.

Selective serotonin reuptake inhibitors

Fluoxetine is the foremost selective serotonin reuptake inhibitor (SSRI) used in the world. It has been subject to abuse in three different ways and there is no reason to suppose that any of the other SSRIs are less susceptible:

Amphetamine-like effect

Two cases of fluoxetine abuse have been described in which known street drug abusers discovered that high doses of fluoxetine produced an amphetamine-like stimulant effect [33]. The first of these initially discovered the effect when taking 80 mg of fluoxetine and two cans of beer on an empty stomach. This produced 'increased energy, talkativeness, mood elevation and slight jitters but she reported that it was unlike 'speed' because she also felt numb and calm'. The second patient took 80 to 140 mg of fluoxetine per day initially but later increased this to a 'handful'. He also experienced an amphetamine-like effect and used trazodone and later diazepam to sedate him at night. Both patients' lives eventually became dominated by the taking of the drug, leading to hospital admission. Neither patient experienced a withdrawal reaction upon discontinuation.

Wilcox described a patient with anorexia who took 120 mg per day on account of the appetite suppressing effects she experienced at high doses [34]. No psychotropic effects were reported.

Augmentation of the effects of other drugs

Fluoxetine has been used to boost or prolong the actions of amphetamine or ecstasy. Limited animal experiments suggest that fluoxetine can increase the levels of amphetamines in the brain and the duration of action of the amphetamines [35], perhaps by decreasing the rate of metabolism. Two case reports suggest that when taken together, dex-amphetamine and fluoxetine may have significantly greater mood-enhancing effects in patients with depression than either drug alone [36, 37]. Theoretically, combining drugs which potentiate the activity of serotonergic systems in the brain will increase the risk of developing the central serotonin syndrome [38].

Reduction of amphetamine or ecstasy side effects

As discussed in Chapter 6, fluoxetine may have some value in the reduction of amphetamine withdrawal symptoms although the human data are sparse. However, fluoxetine has also been used at street level in an attempt to help users cope with the aftermath of acute ecstasy or amphetamine intoxication [39]. In addition, it has been taken in the belief that it will prevent or reduce long-term amphetamine or ecstasy-induced damage to serotonergic nerves [39]. Animal studies have shown that fluoxetine may prevent the excessive loss of brain 5-hydroxytrytamine (5HT) which has been associated with destruction of nerves by these illicit drugs [35].

Tricyclic antidepressants

There have been several case reports of the abuse of amitriptyline [40–43]. This is a drug with significant antimuscarinic effects and the abuse potential may derive solely from this pharmacological property. A study in 1978 briefly described 86 patients on a methadone maintenance programme who abused amitriptyline to attain a 'sedative type of high' [40]. This effect was reported by the authors to be dose-dependent, although precise details of doses taken were not provided. In one documented case, amitriptyline abuse led to the onset of repeated grand mal convulsions and a diagnosis of epilepsy; these symptoms abated when amitriptyline was withdrawn [41]. The patient took up to 750 mg of amitriptyline per day. In a similar case, the chronic administration of 800 mg of amitriptyline daily led to convulsions and toxicity suggestive of overdose [42]. Another patient took up to 2 g per day [43]. The three patients described here were all female and all claimed a calming and/or euphoric effect from high-dose amitriptyline.

Abuse of dothiepin has been reported from Ireland, where this drug is the most popular antidepressant prescribed [44]. A questionnaire of 83 attenders at a Drug Treatment Centre in Dublin revealed that 38 had taken dothiepin for the purpose of abuse. Urine analysis of 99 other attenders showed that 19 had positive tests for tricyclic antidepressants. The total amount taken per day varied from 150 to 600 mg and this was reported to cause euphoria, sedation and various hallucinations (auditory and visual).

ANTIMUSCARINIC DRUGS

Benzhexol (trihexyphenidyl), orphenadrine, benztropine and procyclidine are examples of antimuscarinic agents that have been abused to produce euphoric, and sometimes hallucinogenic, effects. The usual abusers are psychiatric patients who have been prescribed the drugs to counteract the extrapyramidal side effects of antipsychotic medication. However, the author is aware of two Parkinsonian patients believed to have abused orphenadrine. A large number of cases have been described and several good reviews are available [45–48].

As a group, these drugs are not generally available on the street, although cases of abusers purchasing supplies illegally are occasionally reported [49]. These drugs are nearly always taken orally. Patients abusing their prescribed antimuscarinic drugs may go to great lengths to obtain further quantities. They may, for example, claim to have lost prescribed supplies [50], pretend resistance to dosage reduction [51], deny receipt of doses, steal or buy from other patients [52] and even fake extra-pyramidal symptoms [53]. Phenothiazines may mask some of the pleasurable effects of antimuscarinic drug abuse: consequently, patients may stop taking regular antipsychotic medication. In addition, there is the risk that some patients will swap these prescribed drugs for other, illicit, drugs of abuse so introducing antimuscarinics onto the local street scene.

For some schizophrenic patients it is difficult to classify this problem as 'abuse' because the effects sought are not euphoria and psychoactive effects but an increased sociability and contentment [54]. However, others simply seek a 'high' or entertaining hallucinations.

Large doses of antimuscarinics carry the risk of severe intoxication. The exact presentation of the intoxicated patient depends on the dose taken but some of the symptoms are listed in Table 11.1. These effects usually subside within 24 to 72 hours but the diagnosis can be missed because symptoms may resemble those of a patient's existing psychiatric illness. Withdrawal symptoms have been described in some chronic abusers and include rebound cholinergic effects, insomnia, headache, myalgia, various forms of gastrointestinal upset and sleep disturbance [48].

The antimuscarinic properties of certain other medications may, wholly or partly, account for their abuse potential. Examples include amitriptyline (see above) and antihistamines (Chapter 12). Plants with antimuscarinic properties are discussed in Chapter 16. Opioids, alcohol and cannabis can also produce antimuscarinic-like effects and, perhaps

Table 11.1 Potential signs and symptoms of antimuscarinic intoxication

- Dilated pupils
- Dry mouth and hot, dry skin
- Tachycardia
- Incoherence, impaired concentration, confusion, hallucinations, paranoia, anxiety, euphoria, excitement
- Ataxia, disorientation
- Constipation
- Urinary retention

The main features are summarised in a verse:
> Hot as a hare,
> Blind as a bat,
> Dry as a bone,
> Red as a beet,
> Mad as a hatter.

because of this, opioid abusers can be peculiarly sensitive to anti-muscarinic drugs. In the US study of amitriptyline abuse cited above, 25 per cent of 346 participants in a methadone maintenance programme had taken this drug to produce euphoria. The combination seemed to have at least additive effects [40]. Similarly, a case report in 1984 suggested that antimuscarinic intoxication might be potentiated by alcohol [55].

SEDATIVES

Barbiturates

The abuse of barbiturates on the street is now a relatively minor problem. Barbiturates, like benzodiazepines (BZDs), are abused for the purposes of producing relaxation and increased sociability – a mild intoxication. Sometimes the oral formulations are injected for much the same reasons as BZDs. Like BZDs, barbiturates can cause physical dependence, and individuals exhibit both tolerance to the drugs' effects and a withdrawal syndrome upon cessation. Consequently, barbiturates must be withdrawn slowly in the chronic user.

However, barbiturates are more likely than BZDs to cause unpleasant side effects. Even small doses can produce aggression, confusion, depression or anxiety and, unlike BZDs, the drugs are quite likely to depress mental acuity. Barbiturates also commonly precipitate sedation, incoherence and incoordination. These effects all depend on the dose taken. Large doses can cause potentially fatal respiratory depression and this effect is potentiated by alcohol and other CNS depressants such as opioids. In the heyday of barbiturate prescribing for insomnia, this was the usual cause of death when barbiturates were taken in overdose. In the absence of pre-existing lung disease, BZDs are unlikely to cause respiratory depression even when enormous doses are taken.

Barbiturates are less easily obtainable on the black market than BZDs and so are more expensive; illicit manufacture is probably very limited.

Benzodiazepines

There are two different aspects to the subject of benzodiazepine (BZD) 'abuse'.

1. Overprescribing and/or inappropriate prescribing of hypnotic and anxiolytic BZDs has resulted in large numbers of patients becoming dependent upon them.

2.   Abuse of BZDs occurs on the street often by intravenous injection of formulations designed for oral administration.

Whereas the first of these two groups are patients who have been prescribed BZDs for a medical indication, the second group is largely composed of known abusers of a range of illicit substances. For ease of discussion, these might be termed 'BZD-dependents' and 'BZD abusers' respectively.

Benzodiazepine dependents

In 1995 there were nearly 13.9 million prescriptions for benzodiazepines in England [56]. This compares with over 35 million in 1979, suggesting that doctors are gradually acting to combat the problem of BZD dependence. Table 11.2 suggests straightforward ways in which this change needs to progress. BZDs are very useful and, on the whole, safe drugs but prescribing practice still needs to be more rational in many cases. GPs and hospital doctors are jointly responsible for starting patients on benzodiazepines, failing to review treatment regularly and not stopping treatment when it is no longer required. However, as Hallstrom has argued, it can be very difficult to specify why patients should not take these drugs chronically [57]. He suggests that the main reasons are as follows.

- Benzodiazepines are often prescribed to blot out psychological stresses and so do not enable the affected individual to learn how to adapt to stress and thereby mature.
- Patients and doctors can be tempted into thinking there is a 'pill for every ill' and rely too much on pharmacological approaches to treatment when other approaches might be more appropriate.
- A large proportion of prescriptions are made out by male doctors for female patients. If women have an unequal role in society and this is the cause of their stress, then BZDs are not the answer. However, feminists might feel that 'They are given tranquillisers by the establishment to stop them complaining too much'.
- The long-term efficacy of BZDs is unproven.
- Side effects, although sometimes difficult to identify, include memory loss and psychomotor incoordination. Benzodiazepines impair driving ability.
- Dependence is not a problem in itself as long as supplies of benzodiazepines continue; the sudden cessation of drug in the dependent individual is the problem (i.e. withdrawal, see below).

Table 11.2 Avoiding benzodiazepine dependence or abuse – guidance on prescribing

Benzodiazepine dependents

■ Use BZDs only for anxiety or insomnia that seriously disrupts the patient's lifestyle not for minor complaints

■ There are non-drug alternative treatment strategies for both conditions that should be considered, e.g. elimination of underlying causes, lifestyle changes, counselling

■ Warn the patient of tolerance, dependence potential and the difficulty of withdrawal if treatment is prolonged

■ Limit the supply of medication provided, e.g. for insomnia 7 doses, for anxiety 14 days

■ Write 'when required' on the prescription and make sure the patient understands that daily dosing is usually not mandatory for beneficial effects. Generally, intermittent use (by this method or by prescribing occasional short courses) is more likely to be efficacious and is less likely to cause dependence in the long-term

■ Use the smallest dose possible

■ Regularly review the need for medication and discontinue as soon as possible

■ Withdraw dependents from BZDs slowly

Benzodiazepine abusers

■ Avoid prescribing to those with a history of drug abuse

■ Do not prescribe BZDs to temporary residents and be cautious concerning supply to new patients of a practice

■ Remember that non-abusers may sell their medication to abusers, so review all BZD prescriptions regularly and limit quantities prescribed

■ Document known history of BZD abuse so that any other doctor will be aware of the problem

■ Where street abuse is suspected, refuse to supply; alternatively supply elixir which is much more difficult to abuse

Most health authorities or Trusts have produced guidelines on BZD prescribing and withdrawal. It is important that new patients are warned of the risk of dependence and steps taken to prevent it happening. Where practicable, existing dependents should be withdrawn slowly, usually following conversion to oral diazepam which has a very long half-life and thus renders withdrawal easier. The symptoms of withdrawal must be explained to the patient, as these are often very similar to the original complaint for which BZDs were prescribed. Cessation of long-term BZDs is associated with a withdrawal syndrome in many, but not all, patients. The symptoms are varied but include anxiety, irritability, depression, dysphoria, decreased concentration, insomnia, malaise, muscle twitching, tremors, depersonalisation, perceptual distortions and headaches. Symptoms usually peak at about two weeks after stopping chronic BZDs abruptly. Some symptoms may last for months afterwards [58].

Benzodiazepine abusers

The main drug involved is temazepam. Although sometimes taken orally, it is common for abusers to inject one of the oral preparations intravenously. The doses used can be very large. One study cited 3600 mg as the maximum encountered, with 600 mg as the average [59]. Liquid-filled capsules were withdrawn in 1990 but abusers still inject the contents of gel-filled capsules after liquefying the contents or inject tablets after crushing and suspending in water. Often quite elaborate preparation is required. This procedure can clearly have a range of deleterious consequences which are discussed in more depth in Chapter 2. In the case of temazepam, the effects are exacerbated by the irritant nature of the drug.

Temazepam liquid is a low concentration formulation designed for oral administration. It is very viscous. Parenteral administration would require injection of very large quantities of thick, sticky liquid, which is obviously difficult. Consequently, a switch to prescribing of liquid formulations has been advocated as a means of reducing temazepam abuse [60]. This would undoubtedly be a useful measure but might simply encourage the preferential abuse of the other BZDs which are available in tablet form.

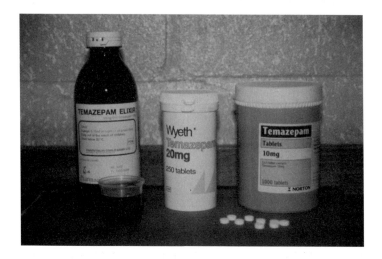

Figure 11.2 Temazepam syrup and tablets.

Table 11.3 Reasons for benzodiazepine abuse 'on the street'

- 'Rush' or 'buzz' after rapid injection
- CNS depressant properties, e.g. sedative, relaxant, anxiolytic, confidence-boosting and disinhibitive effects
- Increase in the intensity and duration of the effect of heroin when the two are used concurrently. Street heroin may be very impure and over-'cut' with bulking agents. Use of temazepam is claimed partially to counteract this
- Suppression of opioid withdrawal symptoms

Supplies of temazepam are obtained by purchase on the black market or from legitimate receivers of BZD prescriptions (Figure 11.2). Theft from health centres and pharmacies may also play a part. Some abusers obtain prescriptions by deception, claiming temporary resident status or giving false names. Illicit manufacture has not been reported. In Liverpool the prevalence of temazepam use in 1994 was estimated at 44 per cent of attendees at a drug dependency unit [61]. In a UK questionnaire survey of those attending drug clinics in seven UK cities, 89 per cent of 208 respondents had abused benzodiazepines and 50 per cent had injected them [62]. Table 11.3 lists some of the reasons for BZD abuse.

Apart from the problems detailed above, abuse of temazepam clearly could cause sedation in potentially dangerous circumstances. The high doses may be associated with 'blackouts', risk-taking behaviour and personality disorders (e.g. paranoia, violent behaviour) and BZD withdrawal symptoms may sometimes occur in the chronic abuser when regular administration is interrupted.

The prevalence of temazepam abuse in the UK encouraged the government to reclassify the drug as a Schedule 3 Controlled Drug in 1996. This made unlawful possession a crime punishable by up to two years imprisonment and/or an unlimited fine. However, legal restrictions of this nature may only focus abusers' attentions onto other BZDs not controlled by this legislation. The seven-city survey mentioned above found that although temazepam was most popular, 75 per cent of respondents had abused diazepam tablets, 52 per cent had used nitrazepam tablets and 35 per cent lorazepam [62].

Chlormethiazole

Chlormethiazole abuse has been described. A study in 1979 provided details on 17 abusers [63]. All but four of these were alcoholics, ex-alcoholics or heavy drinkers of alcohol. Data on dosage are only provided for three patients and each took up to 10 g chlormethiazole daily when available. Seven patients were identified by urine screening alone, so few data are available on these, but the remaining ten patients all showed drug-seeking behaviour of one kind or another – mostly by manipulating extra supplies from GPs. Symptoms of withdrawal were described in two patients in whom dosage reduction was attempted; these were similar to those seen with other sedatives.

The intravenous injection of the contents of chlormethiazole capsules is unlikely to be attractive because the drug is dissolved in lipid. The lipid would break into small globules in plasma from which the drug would diffuse very slowly. There would not be a rapid rise in plasma concentrations of chlormethiazole which would be the effect sought. The lipid vehicle could also theoretically occlude small blood vessels, causing damage to tissues downstream of intravenous injection sites.

OTHER DRUGS

Many other prescription medicines have been abused. Often there are only a very small number of cases reported in the literature. Some of these are described below.

Antibiotics

One report highlighted a case of tetracycline and penicillin abuse in association with alcohol [64]. The combination was said to produce euphoria but this is most likely to have been a placebo effect.

Carbamazepine

Two cases have been described of the abuse of carbamazepine by alcoholics [65]. The authors stated that they were aware of other cases. At least one of the two patients took the drug with alcohol. The dose taken was between 1000 and 1500 mg, which was reported to cause euphoria and light-headedness. One patient, who had abused the drug for at least four months, eventually developed carbamazepine toxicity.

Clonidine

Two cases have been described of clonidine abuse and dependence in patients taking methadone as maintenance therapy [66]. The average daily dose was 1 to 2 mg per day but one patient had taken up to 15 mg on a single day. The reasons for abusing clonidine were given as: an ability to boost the effects of methadone; to reduce symptoms associated with insufficient methadone; for sedation. Each patient was aware of others maintained on methadone who abused clonidine. Side effects of clonidine that might be seen in the abuser include low blood pressure, depression, tiredness, rhinorrhoea and sweating. In the cases described above, both patients experienced a withdrawal reaction upon discontinuation, although the symptoms of this were completely different in each case.

Diuretics

Abuse of diuretics has been attempted as a misguided method of quick weight loss.

Levodopa

Five patients taking levodopa plus carbidopa (Sinemet) for Parkinson's disease were reported to have derived psychotropic effects from taking the preparation [67]. All of those involved were male and younger than the average sufferer from this condition (46 to 60 years of age). Patients reported effects such as feelings of optimism, increased mental power, a sense of well-being, increased sexual energy and animation. However, relatives noticed a range of unpleasant personality changes including paranoia and aggression. Larger doses than prescribed were taken for this purpose – up to 2500 mg of levodopa per day – despite patients experiencing severe dystonias and other movement-related side-effects of levodopa at this dosage. When the drug was discontinued, both the adverse effects and psychotropic effects disappeared but these were often replaced by depression, craving for the drug, drug-seeking behaviour and covert administration. In each case Parkinsonian symptoms were later controlled with lower doses of levodopa.

Oestrogens

Although no cases of abuse have been described *per se*, oestrogens are psychoactive. It has been proposed that women taking this group of drugs for therapeutic reasons could exhibit tolerance and dependence during prolonged administration after the menopause [68].

Salbutamol

Abuse of salbutamol has been reported. In most cases the individuals involved were children. Infants and children may be more susceptible to the psychotropic effects of salbutamol. A study in 21 psychiatrically normal adults revealed no evidence of mood-elevating or dependence-producing properties [69]. However, even in adults therapeutic doses can, very rarely, cause visual hallucination [70]. Brennan reported a variety of anecdotes connected with salbutamol abuse, including a non-asthmatic schoolboy who used salbutamol Rotacaps because they 'made him feel good' [71]. This is unusual because most cases of salbutamol abuse involve the use of aerosol devices. Intoxication with salbutamol and other available medications by the inhalation of large amounts of aerosol inhalers is likely to be caused by the chlorofluorocarbon propellant (ie a form of volatile substance abuse). The eight patients described in four published papers were all from 4 to 17 years old and in many cases a whole inhaler (200 puffs) or more was used each day [72–75]. Edwards and Holgate described abuse in a 24 year old man who used up to 90 puffs of salbutamol aerosol per day and exhibited drug-seeking behaviour to ensure that he had a constant supply of inhalers. However, no psychotropic effects were reported by the patient who had a history of psychiatric illness. The patient seems more likely to have suffered from an obsessive–compulsive disorder [76].

REFERENCES

1. Rosenberg, H., Orkin, F.K. and Springstead, J. (1979) Abuse of nitrous oxide. *Anesth. Analg.* **58**: 104–106.
2. Berkowitz, B.A., Ngai, S.H. and Finck, A.D. (1976) Nitrous oxide 'analgesia': resemblance to opiate action. *Science*, **194**: 967–968.
3. Daras, C., Cantrill, R.C. and Gillman, M.A. (1983) [3H]Naloxone displacement: evidence for nitrous oxide as opioid receptor agonist. *Eur. J. Pharmacol.* **89**: 177–178.
4. Suruda, A.J. and McGlothlin, J.D. (1990) Fatal abuse of nitrous oxide in the workplace. *J. Occup. Med.* **32**: 682–684.
5. LiPuma, J.P., Wellman, J. and Stern, H.P. (1982) Nitrous oxide abuse: a new cause for pneumomediastinum. *Radiology*, **145**: 602.
6. Rowbottom, S.J. (1988) Nitrous oxide abuse (letter). *Anesth. Intens. Care*, **16**: 241–242.
7. Layzer, R.B. (1978) Myeloneuropathy after prolonged exposure to nitrous oxide. *Lancet*, **ii**: 1227–1230.
8. Nevins, M.A. (1980) Neuropathy after nitrous oxide abuse (letter). *J. Am. Med. Assoc.* **244**: 2264.
9. Brodsky, J.B. and Cohen, E.N. (1986) Adverse effects of nitrous oxide. *Med. Toxicol.* **1**: 362–374.
10. Jastak, J.T. (1990) Nitrous oxide and its abuse. *J. Am. Dental Soc.* **122**: 48–52.

11. Sando, M.J.H. and Lawrence, J.R. (1958) Bone marrow depression following treatment of tetanus with protracted nitrous oxide anaesthesia. *Lancet*, **i**: 588.

12. Gregg, J.R. (1988) Nitrous oxide mood disorder. *J. Psychedel. Drugs*, **20**: 449–450.

13. Sterman, A.B. (1983) Subacute toxic delirium following nitrous oxide abuse. *Arch. Neurol.* **40**: 446–447.

14. Brodsky, L. and Zuniga, J. (1975) Nitrous oxide: a psychotogenic agent. *Comp. Psychiatr.* **16**: 185–188.

15. Eastman, D., Hickey, M. and Hickey, F. (1992) Ketamine misuse identified. *Pharm. J.* **248**: 444.

16. Awuonda, M. (1996) Swedes alarmed at ketamine misuse (news). *Lancet*, **348**: 122.

17. Jansen, K.L.R. (1993) Non-medical use of ketamine. *Br. Med. J.* **306**: 601–602.

18. Lingenfelter, R.W. (1981) Fatal misuse of enflurane. *Anesthesiolgy*, **55**: 603.

19. Jacob, B., Heller, C., Daldrup, T., Burrig, K.F., Barz, J. and Bonte, W. (1989) Case report: fatal accidental enflurane intoxication. *J. Forens. Sci.* **34**: 1408–1411.

20. Krause, J.G. and McCarthy, W.B. (1989) Case report: sudden death by inhalation of cyclopropane. *J. Forens. Sci.* **34**: 1011–1012.

21. Spencer, J.D., Raasch, F.O. and Trefny, F.A. (1976) Halothane abuse in hospital personnel. *J. Am. Med. Assoc.* **235**: 1034–1035.

22. Hiroki, T., Teruuchi, T., Kuroda, T. and Kajiwara, M. (1973) On two fatal cases of poisoning due to abuse of fluothane. *Jpn. J. Legal Med.* **27**: 243–247.

23. Kaplan, H.G., Bakken, J., Quadracci, L. and Schubach, W. (1979) Hepatitis caused by halothane sniffing. *Ann. Intern. Med.* **90**: 797–798.

24. Hersch, R. (1991) Abuse of ethyl chloride (letter). *Am. J. Psychiatr.* **148**: 270–271.

25. Siris, S.G. (1995) Do antidepressants have any meaningful potential for abuse? *CNS Drugs*, **4**: 253–255.

26. Pagliaro, L.A. and Pagliaro, A.M. (1995) Abuse potential of antidepressants: Does it exist? *CNS Drugs*, **4**: 247–252.

27. Mielczarek, J. and Johnson, J. (1963) Tranylcypromine (letter). *Lancet*, **i**: 388–389.

28. Griffin, N., Draper, R.J. and Webb, M.G.T. (1981) Addiction to tranylcypromine. *Br. Med. J.* **283**: 346.

29. Ben-Arie, O. and George, G.C.W. (1979) A case of tranylcypromine (Parnate) addiction. *Br. J. Psychiatr.* **135**: 273–274.

30. Le Gassicke, J. (1963) Tranylcypromine (letter). *Lancet*, **i**: 270.

31. Baumbacher, G. and Hansen, M.S. (1992) Abuse of monoamine oxidase inhibitors. *Am. J. Drug Alcohol Abuse*, **18**: 399–406.

32. Neuvonen, P.J., Pohjola-Sintonen, S., Tacke, U. *et al.* (1993) Five fatal

cases of serotonin syndrome after moclobemide-citalopram or moclobe-mide-clomipramine overdoses (letter). *Lancet*, **342**: 1419.

33. Tinsley, J.A., Olsen, M.W., Laroche, R.R. and Palmen, M.A. (1994) Fluoxetine abuse. *Mayo Clin. Proc.* **69**: 166–168.

34. Wilcox, J.A. (1987) Abuse of fluoxetine by patient with anorexia nervosa. *Am. J. Psychiatr.* **144**: 1100.

35. Ricaurte, G.A., Fuller, R.W., Perry, K.W., Seiden, L.S. and Schuster, C.R. (1983) Fluoxetine increases long-lasting neostriatal dopamine deple-tion after administration of d-methamphetamine and d-amphetamine. *Neuropharmacology*, **22**: 1165–1169.

36. Linet, L.S. (1989) Treatment of refractory depression with a combina-tion of fluoxetine and d-amphetamine. *Am. J. Psychiatr.* **146**: 803–804.

37. Gupta, S., Ghaly, N. and Dewan, M. (1992) Augmenting fluoxetine with dextroamphetamine to treat refractory depression. *Hosp. Community Psychiatry*, **43**: 281–283.

38. Brown, T.M., Skop, B.P. and Mareth, T.R. (1996) Pathophysiology and management of the serotonin syndrome. *Ann. Pharmacother.* **30**: 527–533.

39. Singh, A. (1995) Ecstasy and Prozac (letter). *New Scientist*, 14 October, p. 51.

40. Cohen, M.J., Hanbury, R. and Stimmel, B. (1978) Abuse of amitripty-line. *J. Am. Med. Assoc.* **240**: 1372–1373.

41. O'Rahilly, S., Turner, T.H. and Wass J.A.H. (1985) Factitious epilepsy due to amitriptyline abuse. *Ir. Med. J.* **78**: 166–167.

42. Wohlreich, M.M. and Welch, W. (1993) Amitriptyline abuse presenting as acute toxicity. *Psychosomatics*, **34**: 191–193.

43. Delisle, J.D. (1990) A case of amitriptyline abuse (letter). *Am. J. Psychiatr.* **147**: 1377–1378.

44. Dorman, A., Talbot, D., Byrne, P. and O'Connor, J. (1995) Misuse of dothiepin (letter). *Br. Med. J.* **311**: 1502.

45. Anon. (1996) Managing abuse of anticholinergic medication in patients with psychotic disorders. *Drug Therapy Perspectives*, **8**: 11–13.

46. Dilsaver, S.C. (1988) Antimuscarinic agents as substances of abuse: a review. *J. Clin. Psychopharmacol.* **8**: 14–22.

47. Hidalgo, H.A. and Mowers, R.M. (1990) Anticholinergic drug abuse. *Ann. Pharmacother.* **24**: 41–42.

48. Marken, P.A., Stoner, S.C. and Bunker, M.T. (1996) Anticholinergic drug abuse and misuse: epidemiology and therapeutic implications. *CNS Drugs*, **5**: 190–199.

49. McGucken, R.B., Caldwell, J. and Anthon, B. (1985) Teenage procy-clidine abuse (letter). *Lancet*, **i**: 1514.

50. Shariatmadari, M.E. (1975) Orphenadrine dependence (letter). *Br. Med. J.* **271**: 486.

51. Marriott, P. (1976) Dependence on antiparkinsonian drugs (letter). *Br. Med. J.* **272**: 152.

52. Pullen, G.P., Best, N.R. and Maguire, J. (1984) Anticholinergic drug abuse: a common problem? *Br. Med. J.* **289**: 612–613.
53. Rubinstein, J.S. (1978) Abuse of antiparkinsonian drugs: feigning of extrapyramidal symptoms to obtain trihexyphenidyl. *J. Am. Med. Assoc.* **238**: 2365–2366.
54. Wells, B.G., Marken, P.A., Rickman, L.A., Brown, C.S., Hamann, G. and Grimmig, J. (1989) Characterizing anticholinergic abuse in community mental health. *J. Clin. Psychopharmacol.* **9**: 431–435.
55. Drummond, I. and Wilson, K. (1984) Anticholinergic intoxication syndrome: potentiation by alcohol. *Br. Med. J.* **289**: 964.
56. Government Statistical Service (1996) *Prescription Cost Analysis England 1995*, Department of Health NHSE, London, pp. 83–85.
57. Hallstrom, C. (1995) Can GPs really manage without benzodiazepines? *Prescriber*, **6**: 81–85.
58. Ashton, H. (1991) Protracted withdrawal syndromes from benzodiazepines. *J. Subst. Abuse Treat.* **8**: 19–28.
59. Ruben, S.M. and Morrison, C.L. (1992) Temazepam misuse in a group of injecting drug users. *Br. J. Addict.* **87**: 1387–1392.
60. Drake, J. and Ballard, R. (1988) Misuse of temazepam (letter). *Br. Med. J.* **297**: 1402.
61. Shaw, M., Brabbins, C. and Ruben S. (1994) Misuse of benzodiazepines: specify the formulation when prescribing (letter). *Br. Med. J.* **308**: 1709.
62. Strang, J., Griffiths, P., Abbey, J. and Gossop, M. (1994) Survey of use of injected benzodiazepines among drug users in Britain. *Br. Med. J.* **308**: 1082.
63. Gregg, E. and Akhter, I. (1979) Chlormethiazole abuse. *Br. J. Psychiatr.* **134**: 627–629.
64. Reed, F.S. (1976) Antibiotics for kicks (letter). *Br. Med. J.* **1**: 835.
65. Stuppaeck, C.H., Whitworth, A.B. and Fleischhacker, W.W. (1993) Abuse potential of carbamazepine. *J. Nerv. Ment. Dis.* **181**: 519–520.
66. Lauzon, P. (1992) Two cases of clonidine abuse/dependence in methadone-maintained patients. *J. Subst. Abuse Treat.* **9**: 125–127.
67. Nausieda, P.A. (1985) Sinemet 'abusers'. *Clin. Neurol.* **8**: 318–327.
68. Bewley, S. and Bewley, T.H. (1992) Drug dependence with oestrogen replacement therapy. *Lancet*, **339**: 290–291.
69. Menkes, D.B., Fawcett, J.P., Nunn, M.R. and Boothman-Burrell, D. (1994) The effect of salbutamol on mood in normal subjects. *Hum. Psychopharmacol.* **9**: 435–438.
70. Khanna, P.B. and Davies, R. (1986) Hallucinations associated with the administration of salbutamol via a nebuliser. *Br. Med. J.* **292**: 1430.
71. Brennan, P.O. (1983) Inhaled salbutamol: a new form of drug abuse? (letter). *Lancet*, **ii**: 1030–1031.
72. Thompson, P.J., Dhillon, P. and Cole, P. (1983) Addiction to aerosol treatment: the asthmatic alternative to glue sniffing. *Br. Med. J.* **287**: 1515–1516.

73. Brennan, P.O. (1983) Addiction to aerosol treatment (letter). *Br. Med. J.* **287**: 1877.
74. Wickramasinghe, H. and Liebeschuetzz, H.J. (1983) Addiction to aerosol treatment (letter). *Br. Med. J.* **287**: 1877.
75. O'Callaghan, C. and Milner, A.D. (1988) Aerosol treatment abuse. *Arch. Dis. Child.* **63**: 70.
76. Edwards, J.G. and Holgate, S.T. (1979) Dependency upon salbutamol inhalers. *Br. J. Psychiatr.* **134**: 624–626.

12

Over-the-counter products

A hundred doses of happiness are not enough: send to the drug store for another bottle – and, when that is finished, for another . . .

Aldous Huxley (1894–1964), 'Brave New World Revisited'.

Over-the-counter (OTC) medicines are defined as those which are available without prescription from a pharmacy. As is the case with prescription only medicines (see Chapter 11) it is important to distinguish between medicine abuse and unnecessary use. For example many members of the public take vitamin and analgesic preparations indiscriminately. These are examples of the unnecessary use of OTC medicines. Many products are also taken for inappropriate medical conditions or where there is little evidence of therapeutic benefit. Examples include vitamin C for colds and a large number of 'alternative medicine' products. In the context of this article, abuse implies use of a preparation for a non-medical purpose and in order to achieve psychoactive effects (e.g. euphoria) or altered body image (e.g. weight loss).

REASONS FOR OTC ABUSE

Sometimes the abuse potential of an OTC product is discovered by chance while a patient is taking the preparation for a legitimate reason. Increasingly, however, people may experiment with OTC substances to try to find an effect to their liking. Rumours among the drug culture may alert abusers to a cheap, ready source of an alternative to street drugs. Sometimes, OTCs are used to 'top-up' or augment the effects of an illicit substance and occasionally they are used in an attempt to lessen or stave off withdrawal symptoms or for self 'detoxification'.

Certain abusers of OTC medicines are mentally ill and consume these products because of obsessive/compulsive disorder or other psychiatric condition.

SYMPATHOMIMETICS

OTC sympathomimetic agents include pseudoephedrine, ephedrine, phenylephrine and phenylpropanolamine. They may be psychoactive if taken in large doses and probably act in a similar way to amphetamine, to which they are structurally related.

Most of the sympathomimetics have both direct and indirect actions on adrenergic receptors, i.e. they act by direct receptor stimulation and via an increased release of natural receptor agonists (dopamine and noradrenaline). Many OTC cough and cold products contain sympathomimetics and some examples are given in Table 12.1. The preparations are usually taken orally.

Sympathomimetics are typically abused for one of the following reasons:

- to elevate mood and produce euphoria;
- as a substitute for amphetamine by regular users to alleviate craving;
- to combat fatigue;
- to cause weight loss;
- to enhance athletic stamina and performance;
- ephedrine can be used to manufacture more potent amphetamine-like drugs.

A study in 1992 showed that 11 out of 22 intravenous amphetamine abusers had used OTC sympathomimetics in the past year to avoid or reduce cravings for amphetamine [1]. If taken regularly in large enough doses, sympathomimetics promote weight loss by suppressing appetite, as can amphetamines. However, weight loss tends to be small and transitory [2]. Despite this, such products are sold to assist weight reduction in the USA. Large doses may also help to combat fatigue via central nervous system stimulation and OTC products of this kind are also openly marketed for this purpose in the USA.

Sympathomimetics are banned in competing athletes by the International Olympic Committee despite there being little evidence that these substances actually increase physical ability or stamina [3].

Table 12.1 Examples of over-the-counter preparations containing sympathomimetics

Product	Sympathomimetic
Actifed	Pseudoephedrine
Dimotane preparations	Pseudoephedrine
Robitussin Chesty Cough with Congestion	Pseudoephedrine
Sudafed	Pseudoephedrine
Contac 400	Phenylpropanolamine
Day Nurse	Phenylpropanolamine
Eskornade	Phenylpropanolamine
Mu-Cron	Phenylpropanolamine
Sinutab	Phenylpropanolamine
Do-Do tablets	Ephedrine
Haymine	Ephedrine
Nirolex	Ephedrine
Dimotapp	Phenylephrine
Lemsip (certain preparations)	Phenylephrine
Beechams Hot Lemon (and some related products)	Phenylephrine

Increased endurance might be expected by comparison with amphetamines but this has never been demonstrated.

It has been reported that ephedrine can be used to synthesise more potent amphetamines such as methamphetamine [4] and methcathinone ('cat') [5]. In the USA this has led to the manufacturers of ephedrine being required to keep transaction records. Pharmacists who wish to sell ephedrine must register with the Drug Enforcement Agency and keep records of all tablet sales. The Drug Enforcement Agency estimated in 1995 that 100 tonnes of imported ephedrine were diverted into the clandestine synthesis of illicit drugs.

Sympathomimetics themselves possess weak amphetamine-like psychotropic effects; large doses can produce pleasant perceptual changes, euphoria and mental stimulation. One study has shown that 75 to 150 mg/kg ephedrine may elicit similar subjective and behavioural effects to 15 to 30 mg/kg amphetamine [6]. Sometimes the abuse begins when patients taking these preparations for legitimate medical reasons discover the psychoactive effects by chance. In other cases, knowledge of the abuse potential of OTC products is passed from person to person at street level.

Children may be particularly sensitive to the psychoactive effects of sympathomimetics; hallucinations, agitation, nightmares and night terrors have been reported in infants given normal therapeutic doses [7–9].

The potential side effects of large doses of sympathomimetics include nausea and vomiting, tachycardia, palpitations, headache, insomnia, agitation, anxiety and anorexia. In addition, a number of case reports have described the advent of psychosis in association with abuse. In many ways, and not surprisingly, this is similar to 'amphetamine psychosis'. Symptoms tend to be paranoid in nature with feelings of persecution and are often accompanied by hallucinations [10–13]. Psychosis may arise acutely after a single large dose or develop over long periods of time as a result of chronic high-dose administration. In either case, symptoms usually resolve within a few days of cessation, although long-lasting psychiatric problems can occur (but probably only in those suffering from mental illness or with a predisposition to it). Ephedrine has been most commonly linked to psychosis, the effect being seen at chronic doses as low as 125 mg per day.

Other rare adverse effects of high-dose sympathomimetics include tremor, intracranial haemorrhage, seizures, impotence and rhabdomyolysis.

Abuse of nasal preparations containing sympathomimetics is occasionally reported. Agents such as oxymetazoline are primarily alpha-adrenergic sympathomimetics but despite this more specific action they may share the potential for producing psychoactive effects [14, 15]. When taken for congestion, chronic use is often driven by the reflex nasal congestion which occurs upon discontinuation, such that administration must be repeated to relieve it.

The Chinese herbal preparation Ma Huang is prepared from the dried plant *Ephedra sinica* and related species. This naturally contains a quantity of ephedrine and has been the subject of abuse (see Chapter 16).

ANTIHISTAMINES

Abuse and dependence have been reported in particular for three drugs of this class: cyclizine, dimenhydrinate and diphenhydramine, although antihistamines such as chlorpheniramine and promethazine may be involved. The author is also anecdotally aware of attempted abuse of terfenadine.

The mechanism of action is unclear but the antimuscarinic properties of antihistamines become more prominent at high dose and this may be responsible for some or all of the abuse potential (see Chapter 11). Cyclizine also has some structural similarities to phencyclidine.

Cyclizine

Cyclizine is available OTC as Valoid and is also an important constituent of several prescription preparations (e.g. Migril, Diconal and Cyclimorph). The combination product Diconal has proved particularly popular with some individuals because it also contains the opioid dipipanone. Cyclizine has been abused via the oral route in doses of 750 to 1000 mg and is reported to cause euphoria and hallucinations. Tablets may also be prepared for intravenous injection. Parenteral administration may produce a 'rush' of exhilaration followed by general mental stimulation and sometimes hallucinations. The drug is more likely to be abused by those already taking opioids because cyclizine may enhance or prolong opioid effects. Of a total of 120 individuals maintained on methadone by the Trent regional addiction unit in 1989, 20 were found to be abusing intravenous cyclizine concurrently in doses of 50 to 800 mg per 'hit' [16]. A substantial proportion of these patients may have been cyclizine dependent; demonstrating tolerance, craving for the drug and depression or other withdrawal symptoms.

Adverse reactions to cyclizine abuse include antimuscarinic effects, tachycardia, hypertension, disorientation, mental confusion, tremor and fits. Dramatic acts of aggression, emotional lability and violent behaviour are sometimes seen. The general risks associated with tablet injection are also applicable.

Concern over cyclizine is such that it has been the subject of a statement from the Council of the Royal Pharmaceutical Society of Great Britain advising that medicines containing cyclizine should be sold personally by a pharmacist. Counsellors in drug dependency units have found the problem of cyclizine abuse to be a major challenge [17].

Dimenhydrinate

This is available OTC in the UK as Dramamine. High doses of the drug may cause drowsiness or exhilaration, confusion, hallucinations, antimuscarinic effects and vomiting [18, 19]. Dimenhydrinate has been used by anorexic patients to decrease appetite or produce vomiting, and by those who find the sedative or psychoactive effects desirable. Doses used have varied between 600 and 3750 mg per day, and both tolerance and mild withdrawal symptoms can occur. Abuse of the related antihistamine, diphenhydramine, a drug with sedating and antimuscarinic effects, has also been reported [20, 21].

DEXTROMETHORPHAN

Dextromethorphan was developed as a non-opioid cough suppressant. Although similar in structure to the opioids, it does not possess typical opioid properties and probably exerts its therapeutic effect via non-opioid receptors in the central nervous system. When abused, dextromethorphan produces effects which are dissimilar to opioid intoxication. Excitation tends to occur, rather than sedation, and this is also a feature of overdose. One patient likened the experience to that of LSD [22]. Effects that were described by 20 abusers studied by McCarthy included euphoria, hallucinations, illusions, increased perceptual awareness, hyperactivity, time distortions and synaesthesia [23]. These actions begin within an hour of ingestion and typically last three to four hours. When abused chronically, discontinuation may bring about a withdrawal syndrome characterised by sleepiness, lethargy, depression and ataxia.

Dextromethorphan hydrobromide is usually taken orally in doses of 300 mg or more for its psychoactive effects (doses of 1500 to 2400 mg have been used). However, one case of nasal inhalation ('snorting') of up to 250 mg powder has been described [24]. The main metabolite, dextrorphan, could be responsible for the psychotropic properties because it has some affinity for phencyclidine binding sites in the brain [25]. Adverse effects from abuse may include ataxia, tachycardia, hypertension, impotence, dysphagia, diplopia, nausea, mental confusion, restlessness and irritability. Psychosis [22, 26] and mania have also been described [27].

Table 12.2 lists examples of OTC preparations containing dextromethorphan.

OPIOID-CONTAINING PREPARATIONS

Opioids are dealt with in more detail in Chapter 3. OTC products containing opioids are shown in Table 12.3.

Table 12.2 Examples of OTC preparations containing dextromethorphan

- Actifed Compond Linctus
- Contac CoughCaps
- Benylin Dry Cough
- Covonia
- Day Nurse/Night Nurse
- Robitussin Dry Cough
- Sudafed Linctus
- Tancolin
- Vicks Coldcare capsules, Medinite and certain other products in this series

Table 12.3 Examples of OTC preparations containing opioids

- Codeine linctus
- Gee's linctus
- Kaolin and morphine mixture
- Collis Browne's mixture
- Dimotane Co and other branded cough mixtures containing codeine
- Codis, Panadeine, Paracodol, Paramol, Solpadeine and Veganin (compound analgesic preparations containing codeine or dihydrocodeine)

The majority of those who abuse OTC opioids are probably established users of intravenous opioids. One study of 31 intravenous opioid abusers illustrates the reasons why OTC opioids are bought by injection drug users [1]. In this cohort, 20 individuals had used OTC opioids; 16 used single large doses to avoid a withdrawal reaction when intravenous opioids were not available; ten used OTC opioids in an attempt at self-detoxification; five used OTC products to supplement or augment the action of intravenous opioids. Codeine linctus was the most popular product and was named by 16 participants.

The presence of paracetamol or aspirin limits the abuse potential of OTC opioid-containing analgesics because doses needed for the purpose of abuse will tend to cause paracetamol or aspirin toxicity. Observations in Denmark suggest that some abusers are able to separate codeine from compound analgesics which also contain aspirin [28]. However, a separation procedure developed in Glasgow using a coffee filter [29] has been shown to be unreliable [30].

Abuse of codeine linctus is well known, each 100 ml comprises 300 mg of codeine (which is equivalent to about 25 mg of morphine). Gee's linctus contains opium tincture (equivalent to 16 mg of anhydrous morphine per 100 ml) and an extract of squill. The latter includes cardiac glycosides which have caused cardiac toxicity in heavy abusers [31].

Prolonged administration of kaolin and morphine mixture in large doses may cause severe hypokalaemia [32, 33]. Quantities such as 600 to 800 ml per day have been taken (the product only contains 7 mg of morphine per 100 ml). Hypokalaemia probably arises as a result of potassium binding by kaolin in the gut and/or from the high sodium bicarbonate content which can promote kaliuresis. One case report describing a chronic user attributed death to myocardial necrosis secondary to persistent hypokalaemia and/or intestinal obstruction [32]. Reversible hypertension may also occur in heavy users, perhaps caused by the high sodium content of the preparation [33].

LAXATIVES

The majority of laxative abusers are female and the laxatives involved are almost always of the stimulant variety (e.g. senna, bisacodyl or phenolphthalein). Many people who purchase OTC laxatives have constipation because of poor diet and/or lack of exercise – causes that can be easily remedied. This is unnecessary use of an OTC product, as defined in the introduction to this article. There are also patients who take laxatives when true constipation does not exist, a habit more easily defined as abuse. This practice can be very difficult to identify and there is no standard approach to diagnosis, counselling or treatment [34]. Most abusers of this kind tend to have an associated psychiatric illness or at least a tendency towards neurosis and seem to fall into two groups: those with eating disorders and those with bowel obsession.

Eating disorders

Patients with bulimia or anorexia nervosa may abuse laxatives; one review suggested that bulimia patients may be more than three and a half times more likely to abuse laxatives than the general population [35]. Most sufferers are women between late teenage and 30 years of age. They may believe that laxatives will reduce the calorific impact of food by reducing absorption and thus preventing weight gain, although this is obviously not the case. Some ill-informed members of the public who do not suffer from eating disorders may also use laxatives in this way as an aid to dieting. Laxatives might reduce the subjective feelings of 'bloatedness' that many bulimia patients find upsetting or diminish any abdominal cramping [35]. Interestingly, studies suggest that laxative abuse by bulimics may cause an increase in anxiety that dissipates once abuse is discontinued [36].

Bowel obsession

These patients tend to be older than those in the previous group and often have one of a number of associated mental disorders (e.g. depression, dementia, anxiety, various neuroses). There may be an obsession to defaecate regularly at the same time of the day and/or to produce stools of a certain precise appearance. These beliefs may have arisen from training instilled in childhood, from a previous experience of constipation or from a belief that regular bowel habit is necessary for bodily cleanliness. Some may have suffered from real constipation initially but persistent abuse of stimulant laxatives causes a degree of tolerance to their effects and consequently dosage tends to be progressively increased.

Not surprisingly, many laxative abusers suffer from chronic diarrhoea which may result in electrolyte disturbances related to malabsorption and its sequelae. Sodium and water loss encourage hypokalaemia, which is quite common; hypocalcaemia and hypomagnesaemia can also occur. Electrolyte derangement can result in acute renal failure and steatorrhoea has been reported rarely.

Long-term use of stimulant laxatives is likely to result in atonic colon characterised by loss of normal colonic mucosa structure. This in turn causes intractable constipation, a physical inability to defaecate and periodic faecal impaction. Such patients often fail to respond at all to stimulant laxatives and bowel cleansing solutions may be the only treatment option.

SIMPLE ANALGESICS

OTC analgesia is often used unnecessarily. In one survey in the 1960s, 40 per cent of interviewees who took OTC aspirin for medicinal purposes did so for indications where aspirin has no therapeutic benefit [37]. However, abuse, as defined in this article, is rare. It is sometimes claimed that ingestion of a mixture of one or two soluble aspirin with a fizzy cola drink or beer will produce a 'high'. There is no evidence that this is anything other than a placebo effect.

Nonetheless, some people appear to derive pleasurable intoxicating effects from dangerously high doses of aspirin. Two cases have been described by Madden and Wilson [38]. In one of these, 20 to 30 aspirin 300 mg tablets were taken which *'produced an agreeable haze, with a disembodied feeling of detachment accentuated by deafness; tinnitus was 'a gentle singing noise, very soothing'. Salicylism produced a condition of 'isolation, relaxation, protection'.'* Abuse of an aspirin/caffeine preparation was held to be responsible for deterioration in seizure control and violent outbursts in an epileptic who took the equivalent of 13 g aspirin and 2 g caffeine per day [39]. Dependence of the aspirin-type has been defined and claimed to meet the World Health Organisation criteria for drug dependence [37].

Paracetamol abuse was described in four female patients with eating disorders [40]. In each case, overdoses of paracetamol (between eight and 30 tablets 500 mg) were taken to induce vomiting after food binges or when subjects felt overweight. This occurred once every week or on alternate weeks. Clearly, large doses or aspirin or paracetamol, as described here for the purpose of abuse, carry the potential for a fatal outcome.

MISCELLANEOUS

Alcohol

Some preparations contain ethanol in high concentration (e.g. surgical spirit, methylated spirits, aftershave) and may be purchased by alcoholics.

Anabolic compounds

A range of products that are available OTC are claimed to have anabolic properties. These include arginine, ornithine, carnitine and inosine. However, in most cases these claims are founded on poor quality evidence (see Chapter 10).

Antimuscarinics

Antimuscarinic abuse has already been discussed (see Chapter 11) but it should be noted that Kwells, an OTC travel-sickness remedy, contains an appreciable quantity of hyoscine.

Aromatic amines

A toxic psychosis developed in a patient dependent on mentholated cigarettes [41]. Psychiatric symptoms returned when she was exposed to pure menthol. A second patient discovered that Vicks Vaporub and Sinex nasal spray gave her 'a pleasant psychological lift' when applied intranasally throughout the day [42]. Although the spray contains oxymetazoline, a sympathomimetic, both spray and rub contain large amounts of camphor and menthol. Certain Vicks products are also used by those taking ecstasy to help smooth the aftermath of a 'trip'.

Caffeine

Caffeine-containing preparations such as Pro-Plus and Labiton are sold OTC for their stimulant effects. Although no more effective than caffeinated beverages, some members of the public are undoubtedly attracted by the 'medicine-like' format. Large doses have been taken for the purpose of abuse. (see also Chapter 13).

Illicit drug manufacture

Table 12.4 lists some chemicals which may be used in order to manufacture drugs of abuse.

Table 12.4   Chemicals used in clandestine production of drugs

Chemical	Substance produced
Acetic anhydride	Heroin, methaqualone
Acetone	Cocaine, heroin, others
Ammonia	Cocaine
Ammonium chloride	Heroin
Ammonium hydroxide	Cocaine, others
Anthranilic acid	Methaqualone
Benzaldehyde	Amphetamines
Benzyl cyanide	Methamphetamine
2-Butanone (MEK)	Cocaine
Chloroform	Cocaine, others
Diethylamine	LSD
Ephedrine	Methamphetamine
Ergometrine	LSD
Ergotamine	LSD
Ethyl ether	Cocaine, heroin others
Hydrochloric acid	Cocaine, heroin others
Isosafrole	Ecstasy, MDA, MDE, etc.
Lysergic acid	LSD
Methylamine	Methamphetamine, ecstasy
3,4-Methylenedioxyphenyl-2-propanone	Ecstasy, MDA, MDE, etc.
Methyl isobutyl ketone (MIBK)	Cocaine
N-Acetylanthranilic acid	Methaqualone
Nitroethane	Amphetamines
Phenyl-2-propanone	Amphetamine, methamphetamine
Piperidine	Phencyclidine
Piperonal	Ecstasy, MDE, etc.
Potassium carbonate	Cocaine
Potassium hydroxide	Cocaine
Potassium permanganate	Cocaine
Propionic anhydride	Fentanyl analogues
Pseudoephedrine	Methamphetamine
Pyridine	Heroin
Safrole	Ecstasy, MDA, MDE, etc.
Sodium carbonate	Cocaine, others
Sodium hydroxide	Cocaine, others
Sulphuric acid	Cocaine, others
Tartaric acid	Heroin

Reproduced from the Centre for Pharmacy Postgraduate Education distance learning pack
'The treatment of drug dependence'.

Weak acids

Ascorbic or citric acids may sometimes be used to convert street heroin into a more water-soluble form for injection.

CONTROLLING THE PROBLEM

Most community pharmacists are aware of the fact that abuse of OTC medicines occurs [43]. However, it is difficult to know what can be done to prevent the problem or how best to help those that are affected. A valuable counselling service for affected patients ('Overcount') has been established but has no direct input from healthcare professionals. Printing warnings on medicines which state that the product may be liable to abuse or can cause dependence may alert some users to the dangers but will also serve to attract others to 'experiment' with them. By analogy, warnings on cigarettes seem to be a minimal deterrent. Restricting all potentially abusable products to 'prescription only' status is also unrealistic because most of these products are used to treat minor ailments such as colds, diarrhoea and coughs. The prospect of visiting a busy GP every time a supply of such medicine is required, and paying a prescription charge which far exceeds the cost of the medicine, would meet resistance from GPs and the public alike. In addition, as Chapter 11 makes clear, prescription only status is certainly no guarantee against abuse and dependence.

There is a course of action which is more likely to be effective in reducing OTC abuse. Unfortunately, it would be time-consuming to operate and some might take the view that the inconvenience it would impose on so many is far too great compared to the relatively small scale of OTC drug abuse. The situation is also complicated by the fact that patterns of OTC medicine abuse are constantly changing. The course of action is outlined below.

- Continue to educate all community pharmacists concerning which products are liable to abuse and continue to strike from the register those found guilty of supplying OTCs with the knowledge that they will be abused.
- Recognise nationally the existence of OTC drug abuse and establish treatment guidelines for the various forms of abuse.
- Restrict cyclizine to 'prescription only' status because there are non-abusable alternatives available OTC.
- Reformulate all OTC cough and cold mixtures which contain dextromethorphan or a sympathomimetic so that these constituents are removed. The evidence for efficacy of these cocktail

products is extremely limited and any benefits produced are small. The British National Formulary has acknowledged this fact for many years.

- Educate the public that most cough and cold treatments will at best provide only a temporary relief of symptoms and that they will not alter the course of the condition.
- Remove the morphine from Gee's linctus, kaolin and morphine, and similar products because there is little evidence that the opioid constituents are necessary.
- The main abusable cough/cold preparations available OTC would then be pseudoephedrine tablets and codeine linctus. Pharmacies should keep registers for sales of these products to members of the public, who would need to produce evidence of identity before a sale. A similar regulation might apply to laxative abusers.
- The names of regular purchasers should be exchanged by local pharmacies, and patients with an identified problem should be referred to drug dependency units. Further supply to these patients should be withheld. Laxative abusers could be referred to a GP and then if necessary to a gastroenterologist or psychiatrist.

REFERENCES

1. Armstrong, D.J. (1992) The use of over-the-counter preparations by drug users attending an addiction treatment unit. *Br. J. Addict.* **87**: 125–128.
2. Schlemmer, R.F. (April 1986) Phenylpropanolamine as an appetite suppressant: a review of its efficacy and safety. *Pharmindex*, 10–15.
3. Smith, D.A. and Perry, P.J. (1992) The efficacy of ergogenic agents in athletic competition part II – other performance-enhancing agents. *Ann. Pharmacother.* **26**: 653–659.
4. Onlooker (1995) Sorry situation. *Pharm. J.* **255**: 480.
5. Anon. (1994) Manufacturers of ephedrine products must report to DEA (news). *Am. J. Hosp. Pharm.* **51**: 592.
6. Martin, W.R., Sloan, J.W., Sapira, J.D. and Jasinski, D.R. (1971) Physiologic, subjective and behavioural effects of amphetamine, methamphetamine, ephedrine, phenmetrazine, and methylphenidate in man. *Clin. Pharmacol. Ther.* **12**: 245–258.
7. Sankey, R.J., Nunn, A.J. and Sills, J.A. (1984) Visual hallucinations in children receiving decongestants. *Br. Med. J.* **288**: 1369.
8. Stokes, M.A. (1984) Visual hallucinations in children receiving decongestants (letter). *Br. Med. J.* **288**: 1540.
9. Miller, M.G. (1984) Visual hallucinations in children receiving decongestants (letter). *Br. Med. J.* **288**: 1688.

10. Leighton, K.M. (1982) Paranoid psychosis after abuse of Actifed. *Br. Med. J.* **284**: 789–790.

11. Whitehouse, A.M. and Duncan, J.M. (1987) Ephedrine psychosis rediscovered. *Br. J. Psychiatr.* **150**: 258–261.

12. Lambert, M.T. (1987) Paranoid psychoses after abuse of proprietary cold remedies. *Br. J. Psychiatr.* **151**: 548–550.

13. Craig, D.F. (1992) Psychosis with Vicks formula 44-D abuse. *Can. Med. Assoc. J.* **146**: 1199–1200.

14. Shukla, P.C. (1995) Acute ischemia of the hand following intra-arterial oxymetazoline injection. *J. Emerg. Med.* **13**: 65–70.

15. Snow, S., Logan, T.P. and Hollender, M.H. (1980) Nasal spray 'addiction' and psychosis: a case report. *Br. J. Psychiatr.* **136**: 297–299.

16. Ruben, S.M., McLean, P.C. and Melville, J. (1989) Cyclizine abuse among a group of opiate dependents receiving methadone. *Br. J. Addict.* **84**: 929–934.

17. Pearson, G., Gilman, M. and Traynor, P. (1990) Talking point: the limits of intervention. *Druglink*, 5:12–13.

18. Young, G.B., Boyd, D. and Kreeft, J. (1988) Dimenhydrinate: evidence for dependence and tolerance. *Can. Med. Assoc. J.* **138**: 437–438.

19. Craig, D.F. and Mellor, C.S. (1990) Dimenhydrinate dependence and withdrawal. *Can. Med. Assoc. J.* **142**: 970–973.

20. Anon. (1995) Abuse of OTC sleep products, inspector reports. *Pharm. J.* **255**: 536.

21. de Nesnera, A.P. (1996) Diphenhydramine dependence: a need for awareness (letter). *J. Clin. Psychiatr.* **57**: 136–137.

22. Dodds, A. and Revai, E. (1967) Toxic psychosis due to dextromethorphan. *Med. J. Aust.* **2**: 231.

23. McCarthy, J.P. (1971) Some less familiar drugs of abuse. *Med. J. Aust.* **2**: 1078–1081.

24. Fleming, P.M. (1986) Dependence on dextromethorphan hydrobromide. *Br. Med. J.* **293**: 597.

25. Schadel, M. and Sellers, E.M. (1992) Psychosis with Vicks formula 44-d abuse. *Can. Med. Assoc. J.* **147**: 843–844.

26. Orrell, M.W. and Campbell, P.G. (1986) Dependence on dextromethorphan hydrobromide. *Br. Med. J.* **293**: 1242–1243.

27. Walker, J. and Yatham, L.N. (1993) Benylin (dextromethorphan) abuse and mania. *Br. Med. J.* **306**: 896.

28. Jensen, S. and Hansen, A.C. (1993) Abuse of codeine separated from over-the-counter drugs containing acetylsalicylic acid and codeine. *Int. J. Legal Med.* **105**: 279–281.

29. Sakol, M.S. and Stark, C.S. (1989) Codeine abuse (letter). *Lancet*, **334**: 1282–1283.

30. Paterson, J.R., Talwar, D.K., Watson, I.D. and Stewart, M.J. (1990) Codeine abuse from co-codaprin (letter). *Lancet*, **335**: 224.

31. Thurston, D. and Taylor, K. (1984) Gee's Linctus (letter). *Pharm. J.* **233**: 63.

32. Todd, G.R.G., Blair, A.L.T., McElnay, J.C. and Riddell, J.G. (1985) Dependence on kaolin and morphine mixture, hypokalaemia and hypertension. *Ir. J. Med. Sci.* **154**: 409–410.

33. Barragry, J.M. and Morris, D.V. (1990) Fatal dependence on kaolin and morphine mixture. *Postgrad. Med. J.* **56**: 180–181.

34. Eastwood, M. (1995) The dilemma of laxative abuse. *Lancet,* **346**: 1115.

35. Neims, D.M., McGill, J., Giles, T.R. and Todd, F. (1995) Incidence of laxative abuse in community and bulimic populations: a descriptive review. *Int. J. Eating Dis.* **17**: 211–218.

36. Weltzin, T.E., Bulik, C.M., McConaha, C.W. and Kaye, W.H. (1995) Laxative withdrawal and anxiety in bulimia nervosa. *Int. J. Eating. Dis.* **17**: 141–146.

37. Wilson, C.W.M. (1965) Pharmacological aspects of addiction to morphine and other drugs. *Proc. R. Soc. Med.* **58**: 405–409.

38. Madden, J.S. and Wilson C.W.M. (1966) Deliberate aspirin intoxication. *Br. Med. J.* **i**: 1090.

39. Hughes, A.M. and Cannon, L.A. (1986) Analgesic abuse. *Pharm. J.* **236**: 475.

40. Tiller, J. and Treasure, J. (1992) Purging with paracetamol: report of four cases. *Br. Med. J.* **305**: 618.

41. Luke, E. (1962) Addiction to mentholated cigarettes (letter). *Lancet,* **i**: 110.

42. Blackwood, G.W. (1982) Severe psychological disturbance resulting from abuse of nasal decongestants. *Scott. Med. J.* **27**: 175–176.

43. Paxton, R. and Chapple, P. (1996) Misuse of over-the-counter medicines: a survey in one English county. *Pharm. J.* **256**: 313–315.

13

Caffeine

While the bubbling and loud hissing urn
Throws up a steamy column, and the cups,
That cheer but do not inebriate, wait on each,
So let us welcome peaceful evening in.
William Cowper (1731–1800), 'The Task'.

HISTORY

Caffeine is an important constituent of several plants that are cultivated for widespread consumption in the West. The most popular of these are listed in Table 13.1, together with their caffeine content. The tea plant is native to Southeast Asia. It has been consumed in China as a hot infusion for many centuries. The Chinese character for tea is pronounced 'tay' or 'cha' depending upon the dialect. Tea was introduced into Europe in the early 1600s and in Britain was originally termed 'tay'; the modern pronunciation 'tea' originated in the 18th century.

The coffee plant is native to Ethiopia and local legend relates that the first human use was by a holy man who prepared an infusion of the seeds in water so that he might stay awake at night to pray. The plant was first cultivated by man in the vicinity of Mocha in Yemen, the plants having been originally taken from Kefa in Ethiopia. Until the end of the 17th century, this region supplied most of the world's coffee. From the mid-17th century onwards, coffeehouses in London became important centres for political, literary and business dealings. Coffee and tea consumption and cultivation spread rapidly once Europeans acquired a taste for them. European nations, especially the British and Dutch, subsequently encouraged their colonies to grow the plants.

Table 13.1 Major dietary sources of caffeine

Foodstuff	Plant (parts used commercially)	Plant caffeine content w/w	Caffeine dose per typical cup
Tea	Camellia sinensis (dried leaves)	1–5 per cent	10–100 mg (average 40 mg)
Coffee	Coffea arabica etc. (beans)	0.75–2.5 per cent	30–150 mg (average 60–80 mg)
'Decaffeinated' coffee	Coffea arabica etc. (beans)		2–4 mg
Cocoa	Theobroma cacao (seeds)	0.03–1.7 per cent	2–50 mg (average 5 mg)
Chocolate	Theobroma cacao (seeds)		2–63 mg per 50 g
Cola drinks	Cola acuminata (nuts)	1.5–2 per cent	25–100 mg*

* Cola drinks contain added synthetic caffeine.

Chocolate is a relatively minor source of caffeine. It is prepared from the seeds of the cacao tree (*Theobroma cacao*) which is native to South America. A drink prepared from the seeds by the Aztecs was 'chocalatl' (bitter), and was described as the food of the gods.

EFFECTS SOUGHT

Caffeine is taken primarily for its stimulant effect on the central nervous system (CNS). It is the most widely used psychoactive substance in the world. Caffeine produces increased alertness, decreased fatigue, clearheadedness, intellectual stamina and enhanced physical endurance. In those habituated to caffeine, administration gives rise to a contentment, possibly related to the avoidance of withdrawal symptoms but also influenced by the social ease associated with the drinking of caffeinated drinks and the personal expectation of CNS stimulation. Recent work suggests that to some extent negative reinforcement drives the daily consumption of caffeinated drinks [1, 2]. Those habituated to caffeine show a strong preference for caffeinated drinks as opposed to caffeine-free varieties, even when the caffeine content is not known to the consumer [1]. The effect is particularly apparent in the morning because enforced overnight caffeine abstinence produces dysphoria which is alleviated by ingestion of caffeine [2]. It has been further proposed that a liking for the taste and smell of caffeinated beverages is driven by Pavlovian-like conditioning: taste and smell alerting the brain that a stimulating caffeine 'reward' is about to arrive [1]. As with other psychotropic substances, many of the effects are at least partly determined by the expectation of the user.

ADMINISTRATION

Caffeine intake has been arbitrarily classified according to the following values for daily consumption:

- low: 0 to 250 mg per day;
- moderate: 250 to 750 mg per day;
- high: in excess of 750 mg per day.

The amount of caffeine consumed by the average person is difficult to estimate because of the various forms of each beverage and the different methods of preparing them. For example, percolated coffee usually contains more caffeine than instant varieties. If the coffee grounds are boiled during preparation – a method popular in many Scandinavian countries – the caffeine content can be as high as 500 mg per cup. Tea brewed directly from the crushed leaf releases more caffeine into the infusate than tea bags. The various strains of coffee and tea plants also differ in their caffeine content.

Plain chocolate contains more caffeine than milk chocolate. Chocolate also contains large amounts of theobromine, a methylxanthine with approximately 10 per cent of the pharmacological activity of caffeine. Products flavoured with chocolate contain only small amounts of caffeine (e.g. chocolate ice cream has 2 to 5 mg of caffeine per 50 g).

A variety of other preparations also contain caffeine. These include OTC stimulants (e.g. Pro-Plus), analgesic medicines (e.g. Anadin, Solpadeine) and herbal products (e.g. Guarana, see Chapter 16).

PHARMACOKINETICS AND PHARMACOLOGY

Caffeine is a member of the group of compounds known as methylxanthines, which also includes theophylline. Many of the effects of methylxanthines are thought to be mediated via competitive antagonism of adenosine. Adenosine is a neurotransmitter with largely inhibitory actions in the CNS. Benzodiazepines are thought to act as adenosine agonists and it is therefore not surprising that methylxanthines and benzodiazepines have opposing CNS actions.

In vitro, methylxanthines inhibit phosphodiesterase, the enzyme which causes breakdown of cyclic AMP. This group of drugs also has effects on the intracellular movement of calcium ions. However, neither of these actions is likely to occur to a significant extent in humans except at very high doses. Caffeine can also increase the concentration of circulating catecholamines but the mechanism of this and its importance to methylxanthine pharmacology is uncertain.

The average half-life of caffeine in adults is five hours but with considerable variation between individuals (range: 2 to 12 hours). The main metabolite is paraxanthine which is inactive but small amounts of theobromine and theophylline are also produced. Each of these metabolites is subject to further enzymatic degradation before elimination. Following oral administration, caffeine is almost 100 per cent bioavailable and reaches peak plasma concentration 15 to 45 minutes after ingestion. Like theophylline, the clearance of caffeine is accelerated by drugs which induce cytochrome P450 metabolism. Thus, for example, tobacco smoking will increase caffeine clearance but metabolism is appreciably slowed in women taking oral contraceptives.

ADVERSE EFFECTS

On being told that coffee was a slow-acting poison, Voltaire is said to have remarked: 'I think it must be so, for I have been drinking it for 65 years and I am not dead yet.' There is no proven association between caffeine intake and any fatal illness at normal levels of consumption. However, caffeine is pharmacologically active and can produce a range of effects in man. It is difficult to specify the dose of caffeine required to produce particular effects because the amount that individuals ingest is rarely known. In addition, the sensitivity to methylxanthines and the pharmacokinetic profile varies markedly between individuals; dose-related effects are also affected by tolerance, which can develop quickly.

Caffeine-related adverse effects are often wrongly attributed to other causes through ignorance. Recurrent headaches, persistent anxiety, inability to concentrate, muscular tremor/tension and chronic insomnia are probably the commonest of these reactions. The psychostimulant action of caffeine upon the CNS is dose-related but in individuals who do not regularly consume it, even quite small amounts can cause irritability, insomnia and nervousness. The escalation of stimulant effects with increasing dose is illustrated in Table 13.2.

Severe psychiatric upset and convulsions are the ultimate, if rarely observed, sequelae of high-dose usage. Some of the other pharmacological effects of caffeine are also shown in Table 13.2. At regular daily doses above 0.5 to 1 g, the condition known as 'caffeinism' may develop. This

Table 13.2 Side effects of caffeine

Low to moderate intake of caffeine
- Diuresis
- Increased gastric acid secretion
- Fine tremor
- Increased skeletal muscle stamina
- Mild anxiety

High intake of caffeine
- Chronic insomnia
- Persistent anxiety, restlessness, tension, agitation, excitement, panic attacks, inability to concentrate
- Confusion, disorientation, paranoia, delirium
- Tremors, muscle twitching, muscle tension, convulsions
- Vertigo, dizziness, tinnitus, auditory and visual disturbance
- Facial flushing, increased body temperature, raised blood pressure
- Palpitations, arrhythmias
- Nausea, vomiting, abdominal discomfort
- Headaches
- Tachypnoea

Lethal acute adult dose: 5–10 g caffeine

frequently has a presentation akin to anxiety neurosis because the CNS effects predominate. Other possible symptoms are given in Table 13.2.

High, regular caffeine intake can exacerbate the symptoms of pre-existing psychiatric illnesses such as anxiety, depression and schizophrenia [3–7]. The stimulant effect of caffeine may encourage patients to consume large quantities in order to overcome the sedative effects of psychiatric medication. If this resulted simply in the reversal of unacceptable sedation then it would be helpful but caffeine can also antagonise the therapeutic actions of benzodiazepines and phenothiazines. High caffeine consumers who are taking these medications require larger doses of drug to control their symptoms. In the case of benzodiazepines, this is probably due to the opposing pharmacological action of caffeine on adenosine.

Caffeine-containing drinks may cause phenothiazines to precipitate when the two are mixed [8]. The tannic acid content may be responsible [9]. Tea may be more potent than coffee in causing precipitation, although the effect is not related to the caffeine content of these beverages. Stomach acid reverses the precipitation *in vitro* [9] but in some animal studies the absorption of phenothiazines has still been impaired [8]. The practice of mixing phenothiazines with tea or coffee should not be encouraged because of the following:

- If only a proportion of the drink is consumed it is impossible to ascertain how much drug has been taken. The precipitate may discourage a patient from finishing a drink due to unpalatibility.
- The precipitate might settle in the cup or stick to the sides of it so that the drug is not ingested even if a substantial proportion of the drink is consumed.
- In patients taking antacids or drugs which reduce acid secretion from the stomach, the reversal of precipitation cannot occur.
- Precipitation in a drink and its potential reversal in the stomach introduces unnecessary uncertainty into drug therapy. The extent of precipitation, the degree of reversal and therefore response to therapy may vary according to the physiology of the individual, the drug and beverage involved, and concomitant drug therapy. The response to phenothiazines could vary from day to day in the same patient because of this practice.

Superimposing the adverse psychiatric effects of caffeine on top of an existing psychiatric disorder may change the clinical presentation. The new predominating symptoms may not be ameliorated by existing medication. A high caffeine intake is also undoubtedly the reason behind some prescriptions for hypnotics and anxiolytics. Persistent caffeine stimulation encourages those affected adversely to take a CNS depressant drug in order to try to restore the normal sleep/wake cycle of the body. In the elderly, in whom the sleep/wake cycle is naturally subject to increased disruption, caffeine may have more obvious sleep-disturbing properties. Unfortunately, many elderly patients find it difficult to believe that tea and coffee, which most have been drinking for several decades, could be part of the cause of their insomnia.

Many patients with a high intake of caffeine also take considerable quantities of a very common CNS depressant – alcohol. The role of caffeinism in fuelling alcoholism has not been adequately researched. Caffeine is also suspected of involvement in the aetiology of some cases of the restless legs syndrome.

Caffeine can cause mutagenesis in bacteria but studies in laboratory animals reveal no evidence of carcinogenicity. Despite initial concerns, epidemiological studies have not proved a link between caffeine consumption and any cancer in humans. Specifically, investigations have not revealed an association between caffeine intake and human cancer of the breast, pancreas, bladder, ovary or colon. However, such studies are complicated by the widescale use of caffeine and the difficulty of excluding all other confounding variables.

Similar arguments apply to studies of the relationship between caffeine intake and coronary heart disease. Small amounts of daily coffee do not seem to be associated with an increased risk but as the daily intake increases the likelihood of an association also increases. The overall risk associated with coffee drinking is probably small [10, 11]. However, high-dose methylxanthines do stimulate the myocardium so that it would seem wise for those with existing cardiovascular disease to avoid excessive intake. Large amounts of boiled unfiltered coffee have been known for some time to raise plasma cholesterol [12]. More recently it has been demonstrated that as little as five or six cups of cafetière coffee per day can increase total plasma cholesterol levels by 6 to 10 per cent (low density lipoprotein cholesterol by 9 to 14 per cent) [13]. This has been suggested to increase the risk of coronary heart disease by 12 to 20 per cent. The effect is thought to be due to two diterpenes in coffee – cafertol and kahweol – and is reversible upon cessation of cafetière coffee intake. Plasma cholesterol levels are not raised after drinking equivalent amounts of filter coffee because the diterpenes are retained on the paper filter. The same study showed that cafetière coffee raises serum alanine aminotransferase (which is a signal for liver damage) in all patients but that this only exceeded the upper limit of normal in 36 per cent. The clinical relevance of these findings to liver function is not known at present.

Table 13.3 Chemicals found in tea and coffee

Tea leaves	Coffee beans
■ Tannin (10–24 per cent)	■ Fixed coffee oil (15 per cent) including linoleic and oleic acids
■ Caffeine (1–5 per cent)	■ Various proteins (11 per cent)
■ Various proteins	■ Sucrose and other sugars (8 per cent)
■ Theobromine, theophylline	■ Chlorogenic/caffeic acids (6 per cent)
■ Volatile oils	■ Caffeine (0.75–2.5 per cent)
■ Over 20 amino acids	■ Trigonelline
■ About 30 polyphenolic compounds (e.g. theaflavins, thearubigins)	■ Volatile oils
	■ Oxalic and tannic acids
■ 12 sugars	■ Minerals (e.g. magnesium, potassium)
■ 6 organic acids (e.g. oxalic)	■ Various B-group vitamins (especially nicotinic acid)
■ Various B-group vitamins	
■ Minerals (e.g. manganese, fluoride)	■ Cafertol, Kahweol

Caffeine can also stimulate the production of gastric acid, so potentially worsening the symptoms of acid-related gastrointestinal disease in susceptible individuals. Decaffeinated coffee is at least as detrimental in this respect as caffeine-containing varieties, suggesting that caffeine is not the culprit and that patients with acid-related gastrointestinal disease will not benefit by swapping from caffeinated to decaffeinated coffees [14, 15].

Caffeine encourages urinary excretion of calcium but a link between caffeine intake and osteoporosis has not been demonstrated.

Some effects produced by caffeine-containing beverages are not due to the caffeine itself. For example, the high tannin content of tea can cause constipation whereas the essential oils in coffee may give rise to gastrointestinal upset and diarrhoea. Table 13.3 lists some of the known ingredients of coffee and tea.

CAFFEINE DEPENDENCE

Dependence on caffeine undoubtedly occurs [16, 17] and has both a psychological and physical aspect. The former is best characterised by the rituals, habits and beliefs associated with ingestion. For example, many people always take caffeine at certain times of the day (e.g. afternoon tea, coffee with breakfast) and there is a strong desire to continue taking caffeinated substances to maintain/achieve a sense of well-being. Caffeinated drinks form an important part of many social occasions and are part of the cultural background to our society. 'Tea time' and 'coffee breaks' are terms used to describe points in the day when caffeine may be taken but these terms are used even by those that do not take caffeine at these times.

The physical aspects of caffeine dependence are most notably the apparent tolerance to some of its effects (e.g. diuresis) and the existence of a definite withdrawal syndrome [16–21]. Withdrawal is typified by headache, irritability, restlessness, dysphoria, anxiety, depression, lethargy, fatigue, poor concentration and feeling antisocial. Less common symptoms include muscular tension and pains, sweating, rhinorrhoea and nausea. Some sufferers experience craving for caffeine. Headache is the most common feature of withdrawal. Symptoms usually start within 24 hours of abstinence, peak during the next one or two days and last up to a week. In those who consume moderate amounts of caffeine each day, dysphoric symptoms can be observed every morning, after only overnight abstinence [2]. Withdrawal reactions are seen only after chronic administration but is not limited to those with a high caffeine intake. Most users are aware, even if only subconsciously, that the symptoms of withdrawal can be rapidly reversed by ingesting more caffeine. Negative reinforcement may therefore play a part in ensuring continued dependence.

Headaches that occur in many patients following surgery under general anaesthetic have been attributed to caffeine withdrawal caused by forced abstinence.

Tolerance to the stimulant effect of caffeine develops to some extent but, unlike many psychoactive substances, there generally seems to be no particular desire to increase the amount of caffeine consumed with time. Most consumers continue to drink caffeinated beverages at roughly the same intake for their lifetime.

Table 13.4 gives suggestions for making caffeine withdrawal less unpleasant.

Table 13.4   Steps to help reduce caffeine intake

- Educate the subject regarding the potential adverse effects of caffeine and discuss how health may be improved by stopping or reducing caffeine intake. The individual should understand the nature and time course of withdrawal
- It is important to identify all the current means of caffeine intake and the patterns of use (frequency, quantities). Ensure that one form of caffeine intake is not inadvertently swapped for another
- Withdrawal is probably easier if it is not abrupt. Drinking tea or coffee which is gradually made weaker than usual may help. The frequency of ingestion and perhaps the volume of beverage can also be progressively reduced
- Substitution of caffeinated drinks wholly or partly with decaffeinated varieties may help, especially as these have a similar taste and presentation to caffeinated varieties. Again, this may need to be a gradual changeover
- In order not to disrupt the psychological aspect of the daily routine and to keep social rituals alive, the subject should be encouraged to drink something at the time of the day when caffeine was normally taken, e.g. herbal teas (but check that these do not contain caffeine)
- Non-caffeine containing analgesics may be helpful to treat withdrawal headache
- If caffeine intake is to be reduced rather than stopped completely, the subject may find it helpful to limit consumption to certain fixed times of the day, e.g. one coffee with breakfast and one after lunch

REFERENCES

1. Rogers, P.J., Richardson, N.J. and Elliman, N.A. (1995) Overnight caffeine abstinence and negative reinforcement of preference for caffeine containing drinks. *Psychopharmacology*, **120**: 457–462.
2. Richardson, N.J., Rogers, P.J., Elliman, N.A. and O'Dell, R.J. (1995) Mood and performance effects of caffeine in relation to acute and chronic caffeine deprivation. *Pharmacol. Biochem. Behav.* **52**: 313–320.
3. Smith, G.A. (1988) Caffeine reduction as an adjunct to anxiety management. *Br. J. Clin. Psychol.* **27**: 265–266.
4. Greden, J.F., Fontaine, P., Lubetsky, M. and Chamberlin, K. (1978) Anxiety and depression associated with caffeinism among psychiatric inpatients. *Am. J. Psychiatr.* **135**: 963–966.
5. Shisslak, C.M., Beutler, L.E., Scheiber, S., Gaines, J.A., La Wall, J. and Crago, M. (1985) Patterns of caffeine use and prescribed medications in psychiatric inpatients. *Psychol. Rep.* **57**: 39–42.
6. De Freitas, B. and Schwarts, G. (1979) Effects of caffeine in chronic psychiatric patients. *Am. J. Psychiatr.* **136**: 1337–1338.
7. Mikkelsen, E.J. (1978) Caffeine and schizophrenia. *J. Clin. Psychiatr.* **39**: 732–736.
8. Cheeseman, H.J. and Neal, M.J. (1981) Interactions of chlorpromazine with tea and coffee. *Br. J. Clin. Pharmacol.* **12**: 165–169.
9. Curry, M.L., Curry, S.H. and Marroum, P.J. (1991) Interaction of phenothiazine and related drugs and caffeinated beverages (letter). *Ann. Pharmacother.* **25**: 437–438.
10. Stensvold, I., Tverdal, A. and Jacobsen, B.K. (1996) Cohort study of coffee intake and death from coronary heart disease over 12 years. *Br. Med. J.* **312**: 544–545.
11. Marchioli, R., Di Mascho, R., Marfisi, R.M., Vitullo, F. and Tognoni, G. (1996) Coffee intake and death from coronary heart disease. *Br. Med. J.* **312**: 1539.
12. Thelle, D.S. (1991) Coffee, cholesterol and coronary heart disease (editorial). *Br. Med. J.* **302**: 804.
13. Urgert, R., Meyboom, S., Kuilman, M. *et al.* (1996) Comparison of effect of cafetière and filtered coffee on serum concentrations of liver aminotransferases and lipids: six month randomised controlled trial. *Br. Med. J.* **313**: 1362–1366.
14. Cohen, S. and Booth, G.H. (1975) Gastric acid secretion and lower esophageal sphincter pressure in response to coffee and caffeine. *N. Engl. J. Med.* **293**: 897–899.
15. Feldman, E.J., Isenberg, J.I. and Grossman, M.I. (1981) Gastric acid and gastrin response to decaffeinated coffee and peptone meal. *J. Am. Med. Assoc.* **246**: 248–250.
16. Strain, E.C., Mumford, G.K., Silverman, K. and Griffiths, R.R. (1994) Caffeine dependence syndrome – evidence from case histories and experimental evaluations. *J. Am. Med. Assoc.* **272**: 1043–1048.

17. Strain, E.C. and Griffiths, R.R. (1995) Caffeine dependence: fact or fiction? *J. R. Soc. Med.* **88**: 437–440.
18. Silverman, K., Evans, S.M., Strain, E.C. and Griffiths, R.R. (1992) Withdrawal syndrome after the double-blind cessation of caffeine consumption. *N. Engl. J. Med.* **327**: 1109–1114.
19. Hughes, J.R. (1992) Clinical importance of caffeine withdrawal (editorial). *N. Engl. J. Med.* **327**: 1160–1161.
20. Smith, R. (1987) Caffeine withdrawal headache. *J. Clin. Pharm. Ther.* **12**: 53–57.
21. van Dusseldorp, M. and Katan, M.B. (1990) Headache caused by caffeine withdrawal among moderate coffee drinkers switched from ordinary to decaffeinated coffee: a 12 week double blind trial. *Br. Med. J.* **300**: 1558–1559.

14

Tobacco

*A custom loathsome to the Eye, hateful to the Nose,
harmful to the Braine, dangerous to the Lungs, and in
the black, stinking fume thereof, nearest resembling the
horrible Stygian smoke of the pit that is bottomless.*
King James I, 'Counterblaste to Tobacco', 1604.

HISTORY

Tobacco is the dried leaf of *Nicotiana tabacum*, one of a number of
Nicotiana species all of which contain similar alkaloids and which can
be smoked. These plants are members of the Solanaceae or potato family
and are indigenous to the Americas. When Columbus landed there in
1492 he observed the natives smoking rolls of dried *Nicotiana* leaves
which were known as 'tobacos'. The plant and related species were also
widely known to the North American Indians and the Aztecs. The popularity of tobacco smoking spread rapidly in the Europe of the 16th
century. Sir Walter Raleigh was a famous advocate of pipe smoking in
Elizabethan England, a practice that found less favour under the Stuart
King, James I. Jean Nicot is reputed to have introduced tobacco to France
in 1560, his name being commemorated in the genus *Nicotiana* and the
principle alkaloid, nicotine (which was isolated in 1828).

Nicotine is found in small quantities in several other solanaceous
plants (e.g. aubergine, tomatoes) but the amounts are generally too small
to have pharmacologically significant effects after human ingestion.
However, there are a large number of compounds in *Nicotiana* leaves
other than nicotine, and tobacco smoke contains over 3000 different
chemicals.

EFFECTS SOUGHT

Individuals typically begin smoking tobacco when young, commonly in the early to mid teenage years. As with other abused substances, the reasons for starting are multifactorial: a combination of peer pressure, teenage rebellion, the desire to experiment etc. It is claimed that smoking alleviates anxiety and stress and promotes relaxation. There is probably an element of positive and negative reinforcement involved in this response. The positive effect results from the known general mood-elevating properties of nicotine and perhaps from relief of muscular tension. Nicotine can reach the brain within seven seconds of inhaling cigarette smoke and rapid onset, short-lasting peaks of mild mood stimulation are believed to be important aspects of positive reinforcement. However, nicotine does not produce the intense euphoria of drugs such as cocaine. The initial effect is a mild 'buzz' or headiness to which the chronic smoker soon becomes largely tolerant. Negative reinforcement results from the desire to avoid nicotine withdrawal symptoms (which include anxiety). Anxiety also tends to stimulate habitual behaviour *per se* (e.g. biting nails, drumming fingers) and smoking is clearly an habitual pursuit.

Subjectively, nicotine has both calming properties (relaxation, decreased anxiety) and stimulant effects (arousal, increased concentration, loss of appetite).

ADMINISTRATION

Tobacco is smoked in cigarettes which may be purchased ready-made or rolled by the smoker using tobacco and cigarette paper. Ready-made cigarettes usually have a filter which removes varying proportions of the constituents of the smoke before it enters the smoker's lungs. Tobacco may also be smoked in a pipe or as cigars. Nicotine is a liquid which normally boils at about 250°C. The end of a burning cigarette is at least 800°C and such temperatures are high enough to volatilise nicotine so that it can be inhaled. Occasionally tobacco is chewed; those who use this route tend to keep a 'quid' of tobacco in the side of the mouth, thus enabling buccal absorption. This allows a gentle peak plasma level of nicotine to develop. Nicotine is absorbed if swallowed but at least three-quarters of the dose is destroyed by the liver before reaching the systemic circulation. Snuff is a form of tobacco inhaled directly into the nose from the hand. It was much more popular in the 18th and 19th centuries than it is today.

PHARMACOKINETICS AND PHARMACOLOGY

Nicotine is metabolised mainly in the liver. Although several metabolic pathways are involved, the most important is the conversion of nicotine to the inactive cotinine by cytochrome P450. Nicotine has an average half-life of around two hours. Cotinine's longer half-life of 20 hours makes it a useful marker for exposure to tobacco.

Nicotine is an agonist at the nicotinic receptors for acetylcholine. Most of its actions are confined to the central nervous system (CNS) at the doses achieved through smoking. Much larger amounts are needed to affect the nicotinic receptors on skeletal muscle. The mechanism of the psychotropic effects of nicotine is not known. The drug binds to nicotinic receptors in central ganglia of the autonomic nervous system where it can be an agonist or antagonist depending upon the dose. Nicotine also triggers the release of many CNS neurotransmitters.

ADVERSE EFFECTS

It was not until 350 years after King James' pronouncement about the evils of tobacco that the true harmful effects of smoking began to be realised. In the UK, over 110 000 people per year die as a result of smoking tobacco. The majority of these deaths are from lung cancer and coronary heart disease. Table 14.1 lists some of the other diseases known to be caused by smoking. Statistics on tobacco-related illness are alarming: in 1991, for example, it was estimated that over 284 000 people in the UK were admitted to hospital for the treatment of smoking-related

Table 14.1 Mortality and Morbidity Linked to Tobacco Smoking [11]

Cancers strongly linked to smoking
Cancer of lung, mouth, pharynx and larynx
Cancer of oesophagus, bladder, kidney and pancreas

Cancers less strongly linked to smoking
Cancer of stomach, liver, cervix, nose and lip
Adult myeloid leukaemia

Other diseases linked to smoking
Chronic obstructive airways disease, pneumonia
Myocardial infarction, pulmonary heart disease, aortic aneurysm, ischaemic
    heart disease, peripheral vascular disease, cerebrovascular accidents
Peptic ulcer, Crohn's disease, hernia, periodontal disease
Osteoporosis, hip fracture
Cataracts
Fires are an important cause of accidental death or injury that may result
    from careless smoking

illness. These patients used nearly 9500 beds per day and cost the National Health Service £437 million in inpatient costs alone.

It has been estimated that 3 million deaths per year occur world-wide as a result of tobacco smoking. This is projected to increase to 10 million in 30 to 40 years' time [1]. In developed countries about 20 per cent of all deaths are caused by smoking. In the light of statistics such as these, it is remarkable that the smoking of tobacco continues to be socially and politically acceptable. Unlike most other drugs of abuse, tobacco is a legal substance in every country in the world.

Intriguingly, epidemiological data suggest that some diseases seem to be less common in smokers. These include cancer of the endometrium, hyperemesis gravidarum, ulcerative colitis, recurrent aphthous ulcers and Parkinson's disease [2].

Besides the serious health consequences, the tobacco smoker frequently suffers from a range of other more minor ailments, including decreased exercise tolerance, reduced appetite, weight loss, halitosis and an increased susceptibility to coughs and colds.

Non-smokers who are exposed to significant amounts of tobacco smoke may cough, become pale and feel nauseous. Other common complaints include dizziness, feeling faint, tremor, headache and palpitations.

TREATMENT OF DEPENDENCE

Most smokers become dependent upon tobacco to some extent; they also exhibit tolerance. It is well-established that nicotine is the substance in tobacco that causes physical dependence. Symptoms of withdrawal begin within 24 hours and can include craving for nicotine, anxiety, irritability, emotional lability, inability to concentrate, insomnia, increased appetite, drowsiness and headaches.

Various pharmacological methods have been used to help smokers stop but it is important to realise that non-pharmacological methods will boost the response to drug therapy [3, 4] and are also often effective in their own right. Behavioural therapy, setting a date to stop, self-help groups, health advice and group counselling are all potentially useful and are reviewed elsewhere [3].

Nicotine replacement

The most popular forms of nicotine replacement therapy (NRT) utilise transdermal nicotine delivery systems (e.g. Nicotinell, Niconil) or nicotine-impregnated chewing gum (Nicorette). Although both treatments can be effective [5–7], the rate of success is probably limited for three major reasons. The first is that neither treatment physically resembles a cigarette, and the ritual and social behaviour associated with the act of smoking is important in maintaining the addiction. Secondly, simply replacing 'smoked' nicotine with 'therapeutic' nicotine is not an end in itself – just a different source of the dependence problem. Thirdly, neither treatment provides the almost immediate peak in brain nicotine concentrations which occurs during smoking. Patches provide a constant concentration of nicotine in the blood whereas the gum formulation can provide peaks in nicotine levels but they are slow to develop.

There are no particular reasons to believe that any one of the marketed transdermal products is more effective than another. The four main differences are in the nature/efficiency of the delivery system, the strengths available, the support materials provided by the manufacturer and the duration of nicotine release. On this latter point, one patch (Nicorette) releases nicotine for 16 hours per day allowing a nicotine-free night-time as occurs when cigarettes are smoked. This may allow an easier night's sleep. The advantage of the 24 hour release patches (Nicotinell, Niconil,) is that they provide an early morning nicotine plasma level which may act as a greater deterrent to smoking upon waking. Despite these differences the 24-hour and 16-hour release patches seem to be equally effective.

Of the NRT products, nicotine gum has been available for the longest time and has been researched the most thoroughly. The 4 mg strength seems to be more effective than the 2 mg, especially in the heavily dependent smoker. Disadvantages of the gum include side effects: it can cause mouth ulcers, increased salivation and sore throat as a consequence of the irritant properties of nicotine. Some users find the taste unpleasant. Furthermore, the gum requires a chewing technique which is probably not easy to master.

A nicotine nasal spray should have a faster onset time and produce higher peak plasma levels of nicotine than other forms of NRT. Trials with a prototype device suggest that it is at least as effective as other forms of nicotine replacement therapy [7–9]. Nicorette nasal spray is available in the UK and a nasal spray was approved by the Food and Drug Administration in April 1996 for prescription use in the USA [10]. Initially, the spray is used when required, if the subject feels the desire for a cigarette, but the frequency of use is gradually reduced towards the end of the three-month maximum treatment period. The formulation has not been directly compared to nicotine gum or transdermal patches but in one placebo-controlled trial abstinence rates at one year were 26 per cent for nicotine-treated patients and 10 per cent for placebo respectively [9]. This compares well to abstinence rates seen with patches

(20.5 per cent) and gum (18.3 per cent) based on a meta-analysis of available trials [6]. However, more trials of the nasal spray are needed to confirm these findings. One disadvantage of the nasal spray is that the irritant nature of nicotine can produce sneezing, runny nose, watery eyes and sore throat. Because the spray provides more immediate psychoactive effects than any other form of nicotine replacement therapy it is theoretically more open to abuse.

Several over-the-counter 'anti-smoking' products contain nicotine (e.g. Stoppers, Resolution) but these have not been formally assessed in controlled studies.

Nicotine substitutes

Preparations containing the nicotine-related alkoloid lobeline have been used in the past to aid nicotine withdrawal, but they are no longer available in the UK. Nicobrevin contains another alkaloid, quinine, together with a variety of other ingredients. These products have also not been adequately tested in clinical trials. The ineffectiveness of lobeline has led the Food and Drug Administration in the USA to order the withdrawal of such products from the market [3].

Deterrents

Silver acetate reacts with the constituents of cigarette smoke to produce an unpleasant taste in the mouth. Products utilising this effect include Tabmint chewing gum and Giv-Up mouthwash. Again, these products do not appear to have been subjected to formal clinical assessment. The Food and Drug Administration has also recently removed them from sale in the USA [3].

Other drugs

Clonidine, buspirone and antidepressants have met with limited success in assisting tobacco abstinence in small-scale trials [3].

National and international perspectives

At national level, the Government has been loath to be too active in the fight against smoking. There is a significant national and international tobacco lobby, supported of course by millions of dependent individuals. More cynically, tobacco and tobacco-related products generate vast sums for the Treasury each year. When asked to ban smoking in France, Napoleon was candid: *'This vice brings in one hundred million francs in taxes every year. I will certainly forbid it at once – as soon as you can name a virtue that brings in as much revenue.'* Despite the attitude of Western governments, the prevalence of smoking in the Western world has been slowly declining. For example in the UK, 93 billion cigarettes were sold in 1992/3, compared to 98 billion in 1985 [11]. In contrast, it is unpleasant to learn that the number of tobacco smokers continues to increase rapidly in less developed continents such as Asia, Africa and South America, where in many countries there are insufficient resources to meet even basic healthcare needs, let alone the consequences of widespread population self-poisoning. It has been estimated that if current trends continue, 70 per cent of the projected 10 million worldwide deaths from tobacco in 2025 will occur in developing countries [12].

REFERENCES

1. Peto, R., Lopez, A.D., Boreham, J., Thun, M., Heath Jr, C. and Doll, R. (1996) Mortality from smoking worldwide. *Br. Med. Bull.* **52**: 12–21.
2. Baron, J.A. (1996) Beneficial effects of nicotine and cigarette smoking: the real, the possible and the spurious. *Br. Med. Bull.* **52**: 58–73.
3. Haxby, D.G. (1995) Treatment of nicotine dependence. *Am. J. Health Systems Pharm.* **52**: 265–281.
4. McGhan, W.F. (1996) Pharmacoeconomic analysis of smoking-cessation interventions. *Am. J. Health Systems Pharm.* **53**: 45–52.
5. Tang, J.L., Law, M. and Wald, N. (1994) How effective is nicotine replacement therapy in helping people to stop smoking? *Br. Med. J.* **304**: 21–26.
6. Silagy, C., Mant, D., Fowler, G. and Lodge, M. (1994) Meta-analysis on efficacy of nicotine replacement therapies in smoking cessation. *Lancet,* **343**: 139–142.
7. Henningfield, J.E. (1995) Nicotine medications for smoking cessation. *N. Engl. J. Med.* **333**: 1196–1203.
8. Tonneson, P., Norregaard, J., Mikkelsen, K., Jorgensen, S. and Nilsson, F. (1993) A double-blind trial of a nicotine inhaler for smoking cessation. *J. Am. Med. Assoc.* **269**: 1268–1271.
9. Sutherland, G., Stapleton, J.A., Russell, M.A.H. *et al.* (1992) Randomised controlled trial of nasal nicotine spray in smoking cessation. *Lancet,* **340**: 324–329.
10. Anon. (1996) Nicotine nasal spray is newest smoking cessation aid. *Am. J. Health Systems Pharm.* **53**: 982.
11. Wald, N.J. and Hackshaw, A.J. (1996) Cigarette smoking: an epidemiological overview. *Br. Med. Bull.* **52**: 3–11.
12. Mackay, J. and Crofton, J. (1996) Tobacco and the developing world. *Br. Med. Bull.* **52**: 206–221.

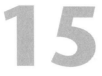

Alcohol

If we heard it said of Orientals that they habitually drank a liquor which went to their heads, deprived them of reason and made them vomit, we should say: 'How very barbarous!'
Jean de la Bruyère (1645–96), 'Les Caractères'.

HISTORY

Alcohol has been available to man for several thousand years. Ethyl alcohol, or ethanol, is produced by the action of yeasts on sugars found in fruit and other plant material. Compared with most other substances of abuse it has a very simple chemical structure. One tends to assume that it was one of the first intoxicants used by man because it is so easy to make. However most of the fruits grown today have been selected for their high sugar content and so the manufacture of fruit wines is a relatively simple process. This was not so in prehistoric times, when sugar-rich plants and sugars themselves were rare [1]. Therefore other plant-derived psychotropic substances that could simply be eaten without preparation probably pre-date alcohol. The first cultures to produce alcohol are thought to have been based in the eastern Mediterranean and Mesopotamia. During the 4th millennium BC they probably fermented dates. The warm climate and the high sugar content of the dates were ideal for the purpose [1]. As the process spread, a whole range of naturally occurring substances were used to produce alcoholic drinks. Some of these are listed in Table 15.1.

The discovery of distillation enabled early civilisations to make more concentrated alcoholic drinks. This process was probably discovered independently by several ancient societies. Concentrating the active constituent in this way enabled the alcohol to act as a preservative and beverages could be stored for longer. In Britain, the strength of alcohol-

Table 15.1 Natural products used to produce alcoholic beverages

Source	Alcoholic beverage
Grapes	Wine, from which sherry, port and brandy are derived
Barley	Beer (hops are added to preserve and flavour)
	Whiskey (Irish varieties may also include fermented oats)
Rye	Rye whiskey
Maize	Bourbon whiskey
Rice	Saké
Sugar-cane or molasses	Rum
Apples	Cider, Calvados
Pears	Perry
Cacti	Tequila (Mexico)
Palm sap	Toddy (Sri Lanka)
Cereal, potatoes or sugar beet	Vodka
Figs	Thibarine (Tunisia)
Dates	Boukha (Tunisia)
Mares milk	Koumish or milchsnapps
Honey	Mead
Juniper berries	Flavouring of gin

containing drinks was traditionally measured in terms of 'percentage proof'; 100 percent proof was equal to 57.1 per cent ethanol by volume. However, it is now the standard practice to state alcohol content in terms of percentage by volume and to refer to the content of individual drinks in terms of 'units' (see Table 15.2).

Alcohol is a very widely accepted substance, even being used as a central part of many Christian ceremonies such as the Communion. It is commonly associated with major events in peoples' lives: weddings, birthdays and special celebrations. A vast and profitable industry exists to supply the public with this inebriant which can have very pleasurable effects but which can also kill. It is not surprising that many younger people feel that Society has a rather hypocritical attitude to abuse of street drugs: condemning illicit substances on the one hand while condoning the widescale use of alcohol on the other. In 1994, the population of the UK spent nearly 12 billion pounds on alcohol. In Islamic countries the consumption of alcohol is illegal.

The 1992 Health Survey for England revealed that 88 per cent of men and 75 per cent of women interviewed drank alcohol at least once every two months ('alcohol consumers'). Of these, 20 per cent of men and 13 per cent of women felt that they should reduce their intake. The survey teams classified 9 per cent of male alcohol consumers and 4 per cent of female consumers as problem drinkers. There has been increasing concern that teenagers may be encouraged to consume large amounts of alcohol by the marketing of several concentrated alcoholic beverages in forms similar to soft drinks, such as lemonades and other sweet, fruit-flavoured drinks. A recent survey of 758 schoolchildren aged 12 to 15 in Dundee concluded that over half of them had been drunk at least once [2]. Another study of 7722 pupils aged 15 and 16 from across the UK revealed that 94 per cent of participants had already consumed alcohol and 78 per cent of these had become drunk at least once [3].

EFFECTS SOUGHT

Alcohol is a central nervous system (CNS) depressant which encourages disinhibition because the highest levels of brain function are most susceptible to it. Depression of the cerebral cortex causes: reduced inhibition, merriment, loquacity, risk-taking behaviour and impaired judgement. As with nearly all psychoactive substances, the precise effects vary according to the dose, the mood of the user and the environment. Blood alcohol concentrations of 0.2 to 0.7 g/L are required for these effects to occur.

It has been shown that moderate daily intake of alcohol can reduce the risk of mortality from coronary heart disease in men over 40 and post-menopausal women, perhaps by increasing the concentrations of high density lipoprotein [4–7].

Table 15.2   Alcohol content of different drinks

Alcoholic beverage	Alcohol content (per cent v/v)	Volume consumed	Number of units
Beers and lagers	2.5–5.5	1 pint (568 ml)	2–3
Cider	3.5–5	1 pint (568 ml)	2–3
Wine	9.5–15	1 glass (125 ml)	1–2
Sherry, port	16–23	1 glass (50 ml)	1
Spirits, liqueurs	35–55	1 pub measure (25 ml)	1

ADMINISTRATION

Alcohol is taken orally, primarily in the form of a drink. The alcohol content of these varies considerably (see Table 15.2). Alcoholic drinks are used to flavour other foods such as cakes and desserts. Alcohol is also used as a solvent and fuel (e.g. liquid metal polishes, aftershaves, methylated spirits). Unfortunately, these products are sometimes consumed by alcoholics as a cheap source of concentrated alcohol.

PHARMACOKINETICS AND PHARMACOLOGY

Alcohol has a variety of actions on the brain [8]. It does affect specific neurotransmitter systems and is not a non-specific CNS depressant as was once thought. However, there is unlikely to be an ethanol receptor; it is more likely that the drug interacts with other CNS receptors by altering their configuration, thus affecting the binding of endogenous chemicals. Alcohol seems to augment the actions of the inhibitory neuro-transmitter GABA and to antagonise certain effects of the excitatory glutamate. This is probably the mechanism of many of the CNS depres-sant actions of alcohol. The effects on GABA, plus an ability to trigger the release of neurotransmitters such as endorphins and dopamine may explain the pleasurable feelings evoked by alcohol. Stimulation of $5HT_3$ receptors may be the reason for alcohol causing nausea and vomiting.

Alcohol is absorbed passively from the gastrointestinal tract – a process which begins as soon as alcohol enters the mouth. It is absorbed from the stomach but passes across the mucosa of the small intestine much more rapidly because of the larger surface area. Hence food in the stomach will decrease the rate of absorption by delaying the passage of alcohol into the small intestine. The alcohol will continue to be absorbed from the stomach but at the slower rate. Peak concentrations are achieved in blood 20 to 60 minutes after ingestion depending on the amount of alcohol ingested, its concentration and whether there is food in the stomach.

Alcohol is eliminated mainly via liver metabolism, although about 5 per cent is lost in the breath, urine and sweat. The majority of alcohol ingested is metabolised by alcohol dehydrogenase to acetaldehyde. However, part of the cytochrome P450 oxidase system also facilitates the conversion as does, to a small extent, catalase. Alcohol dehydroge-nase is only available in small amounts in infants under the age of 5 years, hence their comparatively increased sensitivity to alcohol.

The long-term ingestion of large amounts of alcohol induces certain of the cytochrome P450 enzymes of the liver so that the metabolism of alcohol, and other drugs which are eliminated via this system, is accelerated. Acetaldehyde is further degraded to acetic acid mainly by aldehyde dehydrogenase in the liver. Acetic acid is then either converted to carbon dioxide and water in peripheral tissues and excreted or, because acetic acid is formed by a variety of means in the body, incorporated into the metabolic pathways of carbohydrate or lipid.

The half-life is dose-dependent because the amount of alcohol ingested is usually too great for enzyme systems to handle (i.e. zero-order kinetics). The conversion of alcohol to acetaldehyde is the limiting step. The rate of human elimination of ethanol varies from 80 to 150 mg/kg/h; the average clearance is 100 mg/kg/h.

Table 15.3 Adverse effects of alcohol

Acute effects
- Intoxication (see text) leading to accidents, aggression, risk-taking behaviour and criminal acts
- Incoordination, dulled mentation, slurred speech, reduced audiovisual acuity, ataxia, drowsiness, loss of consciousness, respiratory depression, death
- Flushing, hypothermia
- Diuresis, dehydration
- Gastritis, nausea, vomiting, oesophageal reflux, haematemesis
- Sleep apnoea, inhalation of vomit
- Hypoglycaemia
- Arrhythmias

Effects of chronic heavy ingestion
- Liver cirrhosis, alcoholic hepatitis, liver cancer, oesophageal varices Mallory-Weiss tears (rupture of oesophageal mucosa)
- Pancreatitis, gastric cancer
- Alcoholic cardiomyopathy, tachyarrhythmias (especially atrial fibrillation), sudden death
- Hypertension, hyperlipidaemia
- Malnutrition, weight loss, dehydration
- Peripheral neuropathy, sensory and motor polyneuritis, Wernicke's encephalopathy, Korsakoff's psychosis, stroke, CNS infection, tobacco–alcohol amblyopia, cerebellar degeneration, central pontine myelinolysis
- Myopathy, muscle weakness, muscle pain
- Gynaecomastia, decreased libido, impotence
- Depression, paranoia, anxiety, memory loss, blackouts

ADVERSE EFFECTS

A detailed list is given in Table 15.3. Some adverse effects are discussed in more detail below. It has been estimated that 33 000 people a year die as a result of alcohol in the UK [9].

Acute effects

Acute intake of alcohol can produce a wide range of effects. Intoxication is an important factor in many accidents involving both the affected individual (drowning, falling, suffocation) and other people (road traffic accidents). It is a significant factor in a high proportion of violent crimes and acts of aggression, and may seriously disrupt an individual's social and family life. The behavioural changes produced by disinhibition can result in aggression, fights and other forms of violence, unprotected sex and the desire to use other substances of abuse.

As the concentration of alcohol in the bloodstream increases to about 1 to 1.5 g/L, basic brain functions become affected (loss of taste, reduced audiovisual acuity, slurred speech, awkward gait, etc.). The ultimate sequelae of CNS depression – loss of consciousness, respiratory depression and death – are seen at blood alcohol concentrations greater than 3 to 4 g/L.

Acute adverse effects of alcohol are well known. Flushing occurs because alcohol depresses the vasomotor centre in the medulla, resulting in dilation of blood vessels in the skin. Alcohol can sometimes cause hypothermia in cold weather when cutaneous vasodilation is coupled with inhibition of the thermoregulatory centre in the hypothalamus. Diuresis is a consequence of the inhibition of antidiuretic hormone production from the pituitary. One or two units of alcohol will encourage sleep through simple CNS depression but larger doses tend to cause poor sleep because the somatic sympathetic nervous system is activated as the effects of ethanol wear off. Sleep in the early morning is therefore often restless and punctuated by vivid dreams. Alcohol may cause or exacerbate snoring and obstructive sleep apnoea which also gives rise to poor quality sleep in those affected.

Gastritis, vomiting and oesophageal reflux can result from acute intake of large amounts of alcohol. This probably is the result of irritation of the gastric mucosa, both as a direct action of alcohol and because it stimulates the production of gastric acid. Haematemesis may occur in severe cases. When unconsciousness occurs, death may arise from inhalation of vomit. Arrhythmias are a rare acute effect of ethanol intoxication in non-alcoholics [10].

Effects of chronic use

Chronic regular high-dose alcohol intake (alcoholism) can cause a range of adverse effects. The liver can experience serious damage. Cirrhosis, alcoholic hepatitis, liver cancer, gastric cancer and pancreatitis are all linked to excessive long-term alcohol intake [11]. Alcoholic cardiomyopathy [12] is a recognised consequence of long-term heavy drinking which is probably reversible in the early stages if alcohol consumption is abandoned. Tachyarrhythmias, especially atrial fibrillation [13] are also associated with alcoholism, as is sudden death (perhaps due to ventricular fibrillation). It is likely that those who experience cardiac toxicity are predisposed to it by some means (e.g. genetic make-up, pre-existing disease) because cases of atrial fibrillation have been reported in those consuming a single large amount of alcohol [10]. Electrolyte disturbances may play a part in some cases of cardiac toxicity: hypomagnesaemia is a well-known problem. Women and individuals under 50 years of age seem to be the groups most at risk of dying early (from any cause) as a result of prolonged heavy intake.

Neurological disorders are also common in alcoholics [14, 15]. Many of these arise as a result of poor diet. Malnutrition results when alcoholics come to depend upon alcohol as a source of energy to the exclusion of food: 1 g alcohol supplies about seven calories. Water-soluble vitamins are particularly susceptible to depletion: vitamin B_1 (thiamine) deficiency is the primary cause of Wernicke's encephalopathy. Alcoholics have reduced dietary intake but in addition the absorption of thiamine is reduced and the metabolic activation of thiamine is also inhibited by alcohol. Korsakoff's psychosis is another serious brain disorder that is probably linked to a thiamine deficiency; unlike Wernicke's, to which it may be a sequel, it does not appear to be reversible. Sensory and motor neuropathies and cerebellar degeneration may also occur as a result of thiamine deficiency. Cerebellar malfunction manifests primarily as ataxia and dysarthria. Tobacco–alcohol amblyopia involves progressive blindness and is thought to be linked to vitamin B_{12} deficit. Strokes occur as a result of: alcohol decreasing blood coagulability; emboli arising due to cardiac toxicity; or secondary to alcohol-induced hypertension and/or hyperlipidaemia. Central pontine myelinolysis is characterised by demyelination of neurones at the base of the pons. This can result in paralysis. The condition is probably caused by iatrogenic over-rapid correction of hyponatraemia but the exact mechanism is not known.

The endocrine effects of alcohol are largely confined to carbohydrate metabolism and reproductive function [16]. Alcohol causes hypoglycaemia 6 to 36 hours after heavy intake in those suffering from malnutrition. In other alcoholics, hyperglycaemia may occur for reasons which are not fully understood. This can develop into diabetes. Chronic alcohol administration may cause gynaecomastia and decreased libido in men largely because of inhibition of hormone production at both pituitary level and testis. In women, alcohol may be the cause of absent or irregular menstruation.

ALCOHOL WITHDRAWAL

In the alcoholic, symptoms of withdrawal usually begin within 12 hours of the last intake of alcohol. These include tremors, sweating, anxiety, flushing, confusion, disorientation, vomiting, anorexia, diarrhoea, insomnia and a variable level of consciousness. This can progress to delirium tremens, which may be fatal. It is characterised by severe hallucinations, delirium, violent behaviour, severe depression, hyperpyrexia, dehydration, electrolyte abnormalities and convulsions. Hallucinations often evoke extreme fear. Arrhythmias, hypertension, paraesthesiae, suicidal ideation and hepatic dysfunction are less common but can develop at any stage of the withdrawal process. Some heavy consumers of alcohol do not experience withdrawal symptoms at all.

Many alcoholics have intermittent periods of reduced alcohol intake when symptoms of withdrawal may occur but this usually encourages a return to old habits (negative reinforcement). Full scale 'detoxification' usually requires admission to a psychiatric hospital, specialised alcohol detoxification unit or a general medical ward. Chlordiazepoxide or chlormethiazole are generally used to make withdrawal more bearable. These drugs alleviate many of the symptoms; it is important to realise that their function is to make withdrawal more bearable – they do not prevent it. High doses are used on the first day of withdrawal: 60 mg or more of chlordiazepoxide and up to 12 chlormethiazole capsules. Lower doses should be used in the elderly and in patients with severe liver impairment where hepatic encephalopathy is a potential adverse effect. The daily dose is reduced in a stepwise fashion over the next seven days and then stopped completely. Courses should not be extended because of the risk of adding sedative dependence to the patient's existing problems. Similarly patients should not be allowed to take supplies of medication home with them – not only because of the risk of dependence but because in the (common) event of recidivism the effects of alcohol and sedatives are additive. Alcoholics might also sell sedative drugs on the black market. One US study successfully used chlordiazepoxide capsules on an 'as required' basis rather than via a fixed reducing dose regimen [17]. Patients in the 'as required' group received a dose of chlordiazepoxide whenever an evaluation of their symptoms exceeded a predetermined score on a rating scale. This method was as effective as a fixed detoxification regimen but the 'as required' method, although more labour intensive, allowed individualisation of therapy and resulted in usage of less drug. Chlormethiazole infusion is used when the oral route is unavailable or inappropriate but respiratory depression must be guarded against.

Clonidine relieves some of the withdrawal symptoms mediated by the sympathetic nervous system (e.g. tremors, palpitations) but has no anxiolytic, sedative or anticonvulsant actions. It is therefore not widely used. Fitting can usually be controlled with a regular anticonvulsant (e.g. carbamazepine) or diazepam rectal tubes when required. The anticonvulsant action of chlordiazepoxide or chlormethiazole is often sufficient to prevent withdrawal seizures.

Thiamine should be given to all alcoholics admitted to hospital because most are likely to be deficient to some extent, even if this is not clinically apparent. Thiamine has good oral bioavailability in the non-alcoholic but in alcoholics its absorption can be markedly impaired. Furthermore, if not treated early with thiamine, Wernicke's encephalopathy is irreversible. The usual dose is 100 to 300 mg daily parenterally if possible. Vitamin B compound tablets are of no value in this situation because the thiamine content is too low. They may be useful dietary supplements for general health once the patient leaves hospital because alcoholics tend to be deficient in several B-group vitamins but unsupervised alcoholics in the community are unlikely to comply with any medication. Some alcoholics are discharged on 'maintenance' doses of thiamine (e.g. 25 mg daily). Thiamine should be given parenterally if the patient is not able to receive it orally and especially if showing signs of neurological damage. A patient presenting with symptoms suggestive of Wernicke's encephalopathy requires very high doses of thiamine, up to 750 mg three times daily. This is necessary to ensure that sufficient thiamine reaches the CNS. Very high doses such as this maintain a diffusion gradient for thiamine across the blood–brain barrier, enabling larger quantities to pass through.

Haloperidol is sometimes advocated for the alleviation of distressing hallucinations or aggressive behaviour [18]. However, neuroleptic agents with antidopamine actions in the CNS may exacerbate delirium. Furthermore, most antipsychotic drugs tend to lower the seizure threshold and can cause liver damage, hepatic encephalopathy or interfere with temperature regulation. Neuroleptics such as haloperidol must therefore be used with extreme caution. It is rare to encounter a situation where the simple sedative actions of benzodiazepines or chlormethiazole are insufficient, and many detoxification units never use neuroleptics [19].

During the process of withdrawal many alcoholics will require rehydration and correction of electrolyte abnormalities according to their individual circumstances.

MAINTAINING ABSTINENCE

After passing through the period of acute withdrawal, the patient requires other forms of support to maintain abstinence. Especially during the first six months of abstinence there may be craving for alcohol, often associated with depression. Aspects of lifestyle which help to fuel addiction need to be addressed, e.g. unemployment, homelessness and problems with relationships. Some alcoholics also suffer from specific psychiatric disorders such as depression, schizophrenia or anxiety which may require treatment. Various forms of counselling and support are available but the self-help methods offered by Alcoholics Anonymous remain popular. However, some drug therapies are available which may also help.

Disulfiram is occasionally used to try to control alcohol intake. It usually produces unpleasant symptoms if the recipient imbibes alcohol during the course of treatment. Drugs of this kind are termed antidipsotropics. Disulfiram irreversibly inhibits the enzyme aldehyde dehydrogenase, and this results in greatly increased plasma levels of acetaldehyde if alcohol is ingested. Symptoms of acetaldehyde accumulation include facial flushing, pulsing headache, nausea, dizziness, weakness, orthostatic hypotension and palpitations. Some of these effects can last for several days. The effects of inhibition are permanent and one dose of disulfiram can continue to be effective for up to two weeks. The benefits of disulfiram are limited – not all alcoholics will accept this treatment and even those that appear to accept it may not comply. In addition, some alcoholics do not experience the so-called 'disulfiram reaction' with alcohol or may experience symptoms which can be tolerated; for others the reaction may cause a wide range of serious adverse effects (e.g. arrhythmias, heart failure, hepatotoxicity).

Nitrefazole [20] and calcium carbamide [21] also inhibit aldehyde dehydrogenase. They both have a more selective action than disulfiram, which inhibits dopamine beta-hydroxylase and so increases the plasma concentration of several biogenic amines (which may account for some of its side effects). Calcium carbamide has the advantage of a short duration of action (24 hours). Both drugs have fewer side effects than disulfiram.

Acamprosate is used to maintain abstinence in alcoholics following withdrawal. In alcohol-dependent laboratory animals it reduces the voluntary ingestion of alcohol in a dose-related manner. A derivative of the amino acid taurine, acamprosate potentiates the actions of the inhibitory neurotransmitter GABA in the CNS and antagonises the excitatory transmitter glutamate, i.e. it has a similar action to alcohol. It does not produce intoxication or dependence. Glutamate receptors have been observed to proliferate in the brains of alcoholics, suggesting that overactivity of excitatory neurosystems in the brain upon withdrawal of alcohol may be at least partly responsible for craving. Acamprosate may increase the likelihood of maintaining abstinence in alcoholics after withdrawal. It does not have a dramatic effect and many studies have only assessed effectiveness after three months treatment. However, a study from Austria has investigated the ability of acamprosate to maintain complete abstinence for longer periods: 41 acamprosate-treated individuals (18.3 per cent of the total) and 16 placebo-treated (7.1 per cent) were abstinent continuously for one year [22]. The benefits of acamprosate were also demonstrated in a six-month acamprosate versus placebo trial: 31.8 per cent acamprosate recipients were abstinent at the end of the study compared with 18.6 per cent in the placebo group [23]. Note that in both studies the abstinence rates fell after the active treatment was stopped. Acamprosate does not treat withdrawal, prevent intoxication with alcohol, interact with it or lessen any of the harmful effects of alcohol. A dose of 666 mg three times daily is given.

Naltrexone is an opioid antagonist which has recently been licensed in the USA as an adjunct to the psychosocial treatment of alcoholism. Like acamprosate, laboratory work has shown that alcohol-dependent animals will choose to take alcohol less often when administered naltrexone. However, the two published human studies are small-scale and each was only of three months duration. One study revealed a 54 per cent abstinence rate in the treatment group and 23 per cent in the placebo group but only 70 patients participated [24]. The second study utilised an unnecessarily complex four-treatment group design which had a high drop-out rate (65 per cent) making interpretation of results difficult [25], although naltrexone did seem to be better than placebo. The dose used was 50 mg daily.

Limited work suggests that drugs which inhibit the neuronal reuptake of serotonin such as citalopram and fluoxetine may reduce the desire to consume alcohol. In animal studies, the boosting of central serotonin levels seems to reduce the voluntary consumption of alcohol. In humans, only small-scale, short-term studies are available and these have shown that although selective serotonin reuptake inhibitors may significantly reduce craving for alcohol, this does not always correspond to a marked decrease in intake. The ability of this group of drugs to maintain abstinence in the detoxified alcoholic has not been demonstrated [26].

REFERENCES

1. Rudgley, R. (1993) *The Alchemy of Culture: Intoxicants in Society*, British Museum Press, London, pp. 30–33.
2. McKeganey, N., Forsyth, A., Barnard, M. and Hay, G. (1996) Designer drinks and drunkenness amongst a sample of Scottish schoolchildren. *Br. Med. J.* **313**: 401.
3. Miller, P.McC., Plant, M. (1996) Drinking, smoking and illicit drug use among 15 and 16 year olds in the United Kingdom. *Br. Med. J.* **313**: 394–397.
4. Kemm, J. (1995) How much alcohol can people drink without harming themselves? *Medicine*, **23**: 45–46
5. Rimm, E.B., Klatsky, A., Grobbee, D. and Stampfer, M.J. (1996) Review of moderate alcohol consumption and reduced risk of coronary heart disease: is the effect due to beer, wine or spirits? *Br. Med. J.* **312**: 731–736.
6. Hein, H.O., Suadicani, P. and Gyntelberg, F. (1996) Alcohol consumption, serum low density lipoprotein cholesterol concentration, and risk of ischaemic heart disease: six year follow up in the Copenhagen study. *Br. Med. J.* **312**: 736–741.
7. Jackson, R. and Beaglehole, R. (1995) Alcohol consumption guidelines: relative safety *vs* absolute risks and benefits (commentary). *Lancet*, **346**: 716.
8. Nutt, D.J. and Peters, T.J. (1994) Alcohol: the drug. *Br. Med. Bull.* **50(1)**: 5–17.
9. Godfrey, C. and Maynard, A. (1992) A health strategy for alcohol: setting targets and choosing policies. YARTIC Occasional Paper 1, Centre for Health Economics, York, UK.
10. Thornton, J.R. (1984) Atrial fibrillation in healthy non-alcoholic people after an alcoholic binge. *Lancet*, **ii**: 1013–1014.
11. Brunt, P.W. and McGee, J.O'D. (1995) Chronic alcohol abuse: alimentary tract, pancreas and liver. *Medicine*, **23**: 54–60.
12. Preedy, V.R., Atkinson, L.M., Richardson, P.J. and Peters, T.J. (1993) Mechanisms of ethanol-induced cardiac damage. *Br. Heart J.* **69**: 197–200.
13. Koskinen, P. and Kupari, M. (1992) Alcohol and cardiac arrhythmias. *Br. Med. J.* **304**: 1394.
14. Watson, J.D.G., Kril, J.J. and Lennane, K.J. (1995) Neurological, neuropathological and psychiatric aspects of alcoholism. *Medicine*, **23**: 61–65.

15. Charness, M.E., Simon, R.P. and Greenberg, D.A. (1989) Ethanol and the nervous system. *N. Engl. J. Med.* **321**: 442–454.

16. Anon. (1994) Alcohol and hormones. *Alcohol Alert,* **26**: 1–4.

17. Saitz, R., Mayo-Smith, M.F., Roberts, M.S., Redmond, H.A., Bernard, D.R. and Calkins, D.R. (1994) Individualized treatment for alcohol withdrawal. *J. Am. Med. Assoc.* **272**: 519–523.

18. Anon. (1991) Alcohol problems in the general hospital, *Drugs Ther. Bull.* **29**: 69–71.

19. Gillman, M.A. and Lichtigfeld, F.J. (1990) The drug management of severe alcohol withdrawal syndrome. *Postgrad. Med. J.* **66**: 1005–1009.

20. Stockwell, T., Sutherland, G. and Edwards, G. (1984) The impact of a new alcohol sensitizing agent (nitrefazole) on craving in severely dependent alcoholics. *Br. J. Addict.* **79**: 403–409.

21. Peachey, J.E., Annis, H.M., Bornstein, E.R., Sykora, K., Maglana, S.M. and Shamai, S. (1989) Calcium carbamide in alcoholism treatment part 1: a placebo-controlled, double-blind clinical trial of short-term efficacy. *Br. J. Addict.* **84**: 877–887.

22. Whitworth, A.B., Fischer, F., Lesch, O.M. *et al.* (1996) Comparison of acamprosate and placebo in long-term treatment of alcohol dependence. *Lancet,* **347**: 1438–1442.

23. Paille, F.M., Guelfi, J.D., Perkins, A.C., Royer, R.J., Steu, L. and Parot, P. (1995) Double-blind randomized multicentre trial of acamprosate in maintaining abstinence from alcohol. *Alcohol Alcoholism,* **30**: 239–247.

24. Volpicelli, J.R., Alterman, A.J., Hayashida, M. and O'Brien, C.P. (1992) Naltrexone in the treatment of alcohol dependence. *Arch. Gen. Psychiatr.* **49**: 876–880.

25. O'Malley, S.S., Jaffe, A.J., Chang, G., Schottenfield, R.S., Meyer, R.E. and Rounsaville, B. (1992) Naltrexone and coping skills therapy for alcohol dependence. A controlled study. *Arch. Gen. Psychiatr.* **49**: 881–887.

26. Lejoyeux, M. (1996) Use of serotonin (5-hydroxytryptamine) reuptake inhibitors in the treatment of alcoholism. *Alcohol Alcoholism,* **31 (suppl. 1)**: 69–75.

16

Plants

*And the Lord God took the man, and put him into the
Garden of Eden to dress it and to keep it.*

The Bible, Genesis 2: v.15.

Deliberate self-intoxication with plant material is an ancient human
practice. Mescaline-containing plants have been used by the people of
Central America for at least 10 000 years and nicotine abuse has been
identified from Sudanese remains of 5000 BC. Cannabis was known to
the Chinese in 4000 BC as well as to the ancient Egyptians. Tobacco,
tea, coffee and cannabis are the most conspicuous psychotropic plant
materials that are still widely used. These have been the subject of earlier
chapters in this book.

Many street drugs have strong links with the plant kingdom.
Cannabis and cocaine are clearly derived directly from plants (*Cannabis
sativa* and *Erythroxylum coca* respectively). Opioids are all ultimately
analogues of the morphine found in the opium poppy, *Papaver
somniferum*. LSD is a modified form of the inactive lysergic acid found
in the rye fungus or ergot (*Claviceps purpurea*), although there are many
other LSD-like compounds found in nature which are psychoactive.
Several examples of amphetamine-like substances have also been isolated
from plants.

Some of the plants that are abused throughout the world today
are considered below and their similarities with more well known drugs
of abuse highlighted.

HALLUCINOGENIC MUSHROOMS

There are 12 species of fungi native to Great Britain which contain
psychoactive compounds. Collectively, they are often referred to as

'magic mushrooms' but only two species are commonly abused: *Amanita muscaria* (fly agaric) and *Psilocybe semilanceata* (liberty cap). The extent of abuse is very difficult to quantify but a survey of 3075 university students from around the UK in 1996 found that 16 per cent had used hallucinogenic mushrooms on at least one occasion [1]. Only 0.4 per cent of the 3075 used them regularly (at least once a week).

One of the main concerns that arise when wild mushrooms are abused is that novices may incorrectly identify them and consume other more poisonous varieties. *Amanita phalloides* and *A. virosa*, for example, are extremely toxic.

Those purchasing mushrooms on the black market may be sold inactive harmless forms or varieties that have been injected with LSD, phencyclidine or other psychoactive substances. Several studies have shown that only a small percentage of mushrooms offered for sale are true hallucinogenic species.

The legal position with regard to mushrooms is not straightforward in the UK. Although the active constituents are controlled under the Misuse of Drugs Act, this does not necessarily apply to the whole mushrooms. Picking or owning mushrooms is therefore not always illegal. However, preparing them to be eaten (cutting up, cooking, etc.) is an offence and in 1990 a case was brought successfully against individuals who had clearly intended to supply mushrooms on a large scale to others for the purpose of abuse.

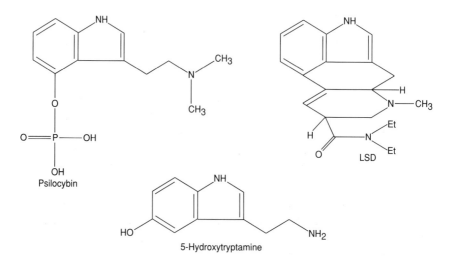

Figure 16.1 Similarity of psilocybin structure to 5-hydroxytryptamine and LSD.

Psilocybe species

Psilocybe species [2–4] contain two hallucinogenic alkaloids: psilocybin and psilocin. Both have an indole-based structure reminiscent of 5-hydroxytryptamine and LSD (see Figure 16.1). However, these alkaloids have only 0.5 to 1 per cent of the psychotropic activity of LSD. Fungal species with the same psychoactive constituents are found in Central America and were used by the Aztecs as part of their religious rites. The British species, *Psilocybe semilanceata*, is commonly found in damp areas of open places such as parks, fields and meadows. It grows from late summer to the end of autumn and the yellow to buff-coloured mushrooms are up to 10 cm high. Related species such as *P. coprophila* and *P. montana* are more rare but contain the same alkaloids.

The fresh mushrooms may be eaten raw or cooked. They may be dried or frozen for later use or made into a hot infusion. Intravenous injection of prepared fungal extracts has been reported but is probably extremely rare. The amount ingested to some extent determines the effects produced. A small number of mushrooms (two to four) may be enough to promote relaxation and/or mild euphoria but some 20 to 30 are usually required to produce a full psychedelic experience. This is characterised by feelings of relaxation, time distortions, euphoria, hallucinations and sometimes synaesthesia (hearing colours, seeing sounds, etc.).

In many respects, the effects of *Psilocybe* intoxication are very similar to those of LSD except that LSD does not tend to cause euphoria. As with many psychoactive substances, the desired experience is often preceded by sympathomimetic effects such as flushing, tachycardia and dry mouth. If an infusion is consumed, the effects can begin within five minutes of ingestion but if the mushrooms are eaten, at least half an hour is required. The effects can sometimes be delayed by a few hours if the mushrooms are not broken up into small enough pieces and if they are eaten with a meal. The usual duration of the psychedelic experience is four to eight hours, and it is often followed by drowsiness and sleep. 'Flashbacks' have been reported.

As with all psychoactive drugs of abuse, a bad 'trip' may occur at any time and may include panic reactions, severe agitation, frightening illusions or hallucinations and acute psychosis. Other adverse reactions include vomiting, abdominal cramps, paraesthesia, ataxia and convulsions. Intravenous use has resulted in cyanosis, recurrent vomiting and severe 'flu-like' symptoms.

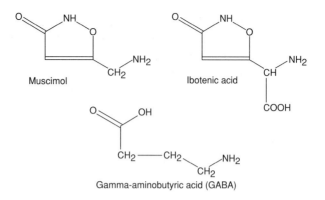

Muscimol

Ibotenic acid

Gamma-aminobutyric acid (GABA)

Figure 16.2 Ibotenic acid and muscimol – probably GABA agonists.

Amanita muscaria [2]

Amanita muscaria also has two psychoactive constituents: ibotenic acid and muscimol (Figure 16.2). It too has a long history of abuse. The mushrooms have a very distinctive appearance. The cap is round and red with small white flecks on the upper surface, and a white under-side: the typical 'toadstool' of childhood fiction (Figure 16.3).

These mushrooms are usually found in September in woods or other areas under the shelter of trees. They generally occur singly but are sometimes in small groups.

Unlike *Psilocybe* alkaloids, which interact with the central 5-hydroxy-tryptamine (5HT) system, the active constituents of *A. muscaria* seem

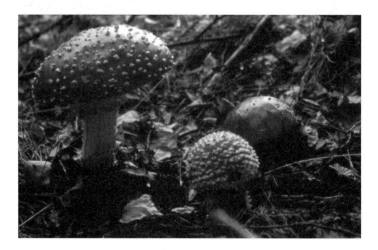

Figure 16.3 *Amanita muscaria,* fly agaric.

to have more depressant actions on the central nervous system. Both muscinol and ibotenic acid probably act as agonists of the central inhibitory neurotransmitter, GABA (gamma-aminobutyric acid). The dose required can only be determined by experience because the mushrooms vary so greatly in size. A 'trip' often starts with feelings of drowsiness but may then progress to confusion, delirium, sensory delusions, slurred speech, incoordination and sometimes euphoria. Headaches, vomiting and convulsions have also been described. Often this is followed by a deep sleep which may include vivid dreams.

NUTMEG

The hard kernel contained within the fruit of *Myristica fragrans* is commonly called nutmeg (Figure 16.4). The aromatic ethers contained within it – myristicin and elimicin – are structurally related to amphetamine derivatives such as ecstasy. Human metabolism may actually introduce the side chain amino group necessary for true amphetamine status (see Figure 16.5). After administration it takes some hours for psychotropic actions to develop, suggesting that metabolic conversion is needed for activation. Psychoactive effects usually begin within six hours.

Nutmeg is ground to a fine powder before use. It is then usually ingested mixed with a drink but it can be smoked, inhaled nasally or vaporised. As little as one nutmeg may be enough to provoke euphoria,

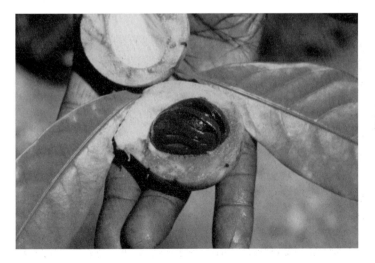

Figure 16.4 Nutmeg. The central kernel is nutmeg and the red surrounding arillus is mace.

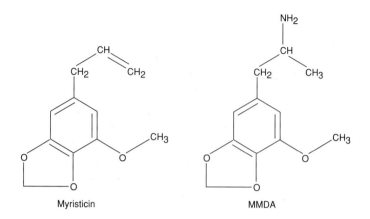

Figure 16.5 Myristicin may be converted to
2-methoxy-3,4-methylenedioxyamphetamine (MMDA) *in vivo*.

illusions and hallucinations. Reports of nutmeg intoxication commonly describe severe headaches, tingling and numbness of the extremities, and nausea or vomiting. This may be accompanied by antimuscarinic-like reactions (dry mouth, flushing, tachycardia etc.) and unpleasant psychotomimetic effects (agitation, hallucinations, sense of impending death etc.). Other common acute effects include dizziness, drowsiness and confusion. Usually the actions of nutmeg last for about 24 hours but sometimes longer and, as with synthetic amphetamine derivatives, the abuser often feels very tired afterwards.

There is a great variation in the response to nutmeg. This is probably because the psychotropic elements are contained within the volatile oil of the kernel, and oil content varies markedly according to age and storage conditions. Serious side effects have been occasionally reported and several cases of nutmeg abuse requiring medical attention have been described [2, 5–8]. Severe reactions have included convulsions, hypotension and shock. A case of chronic psychosis linked to long-term nutmeg administration has also been documented [5]. Interestingly, the patient's condition was complicated by polydipsia and hyponatraemia secondary to water overload; these symptoms have also been described in ecstasy users (see Chapter 8).

Nutmeg abuse is probably uncommon through ignorance and because preparation and administration is awkward. The effects are slow to onset and can be less subjectively pleasant than those associated with many alternative psychoactive substances. Other plants, such as parsley and carrots, contain myristicin but not in large enough quantities to be readily abused.

KHAT

Khat or qat is the common name for *Catha edulis*, an evergreen shrub with a native range extending from north and east Africa (Ethiopia, Kenya, Somalia) through Yemen to Afghanistan. The leaves are usually chewed but are sometimes smoked or prepared as an infusion. The two principal active constituents are cathine ([+]-norpseudoephedrine) and cathinone, which have structures and psychostimulant effects similar to amphetamines [9] (see Figure 16.6). Cathinone is the keto-analogue of cathine and is the constituent primarily responsible for the psychoactive effects sought by users. Khat reduces tiredness and hunger, and causes heightened alertness, sociability and creativity, as well as euphoria and hallucinations.

Reported side effects [9–11] are also similar to amphetamines and include anorexia, insomnia, sympathomimetic reactions, 'bad trips', mania, psychosis [11–13], hypertension, arrhythmias and hyperthermia. Post-abuse lethargy, tiredness or depression may occur.

Chronic use can be associated with physical dependence. Withdrawal and subsequent abstinence from khat has been successfully managed with bromocriptine [14]. There may be a link between chronic khat chewing and certain oral cancers [15]. In addition, khat tends to stain teeth brown and cause constipation, stomatitis and gastritis due to the tannins contained in the plant. Recent studies have also shown that chronic use can decrease semen volume, the proportion of normal sperm, sperm count and motility [16].

Cathinone is very labile and the content in leaves diminishes rapidly after collection, so for maximum effect leaves must be fresh. In the past this has limited the spread of khat abuse but during the 1980s exportation of leaves by air began and this has enabled immigrants in

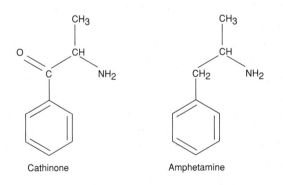

Cathinone   Amphetamine

Figure 16.6 Cathinone, from khat, is related to amphetamine.

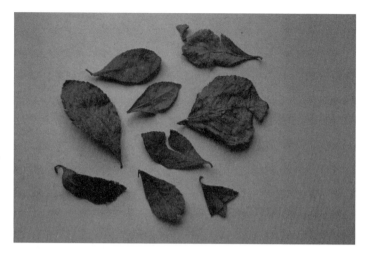

Figure 16.7 Dried leaves of khat.

the UK, much of Europe and the USA to continue their traditional habit [17]. The leaves are illustrated in Figure 16.7. Importation of khat is illegal in France and Switzerland. In many of the countries of origin, khat is the main social drug of abuse – tobacco and alcohol being less freely available or socially acceptable [10]. In the UK, the active constituents of khat are controlled by the Misuse of Drugs Act but khat itself is not. As with 'magic mushrooms' therefore, possession and handling of plant material is not technically an offence but preparing the leaves to be consumed is considered illegal.

MORNING GLORY

The species of morning glory with hallucinogenic potential is *Ipomoea tricolor*, which is native to Central and South America. It is also known as ololiuqui. The European morning glory (*Ipomoea purpurea*) does not contain psychoactive alkaloids [18]. However, the seeds of *I. tricolor* can be purchased from gardening shops. The principal active constituent is D-lysergic acid amide (ergine), which is closely related in structure and actions to LSD. At least 200 seeds are needed to produce a 'trip'. The seeds are ground up and then eaten or prepared into an infusion. The subjective effects are similar to those of LSD.

CAFFEINE-CONTAINING PLANTS

Several plants that are used for psychotropic effects contain caffeine as the principal active constituent. Some of the plants involved are listed

Table 16.1 Plants containing caffeine

■ Coffee	*Coffea arabica* (and other species)
■ Tea	*Camellia sinensis*
■ Cola	*Cola acuminata* and *C. nitida*
■ Mate	*Ilex paraguensis*
■ Guarana	*Paullinia cupana* (var. *sorbilis*)

in Table 16.1. Guarana is a popular product, sold in health food shops and pharmacies, which contains much larger amounts of caffeine than any of the other plants listed. Some abusers of amphetamine and ecstasy claim that it helps them to cope with the depressant and fatiguing aftermath of a 'trip'. This is not surprising because both amphetamines and caffeine are central nervous system (CNS) stimulants. Other than the effects attributable to caffeine, claims that guarana has any special psychoactive or energy-boosting properties are unfounded [19, 20]. However, it is known that guarana may have a more prolonged stimulant effect than other caffeine-containing plants because the caffeine is extensively bound to tannins which only release the alkaloid slowly in the human gut [21]. The high tannin content can give rise to constipation if guarana is taken regularly.

The chewing of cola (kola) nuts is very popular in West Africa. Towards the end of the 19th century, an extract of cola was mixed with an extract of the coca plant to form the drink Coca-Cola. It thus originally contained a mixture of caffeine and cocaine. The modern formula does not utilise drugs extracted from plants: synthetic caffeine is used and cocaine is no longer included!

POTATO FAMILY

The plants of the potato family (Solanaceae) are economically and pharmacologically very important. The tobacco plant (*Nicotiana tabacum*) is the only one widely abused today. However, historically the solanaceous plants were important substances of abuse in Europe. The four main plants involved were: mandrake (*Mandragora officinarum*), henbane (*Hyoscyamus niger*), deadly nightshade (*Atropa belladonna*) and the thorn apple (*Datura stramonium*).

All of these species contain the antimuscarinic compounds hyoscyamine, hyoscine and atropine. Antimuscarinic drugs are known to have the potential for abuse and are sometimes taken for his purpose even today (see Chapter 10). The use of the plants above – the so-called 'hexing herbs' – has been associated with witchcraft. Mixtures of them were formed into an ointment and topical application is known to produce a range of effects including sensations of flying through the air and illusions of human transformation into animals – typical features of witch folklore. Witches sometimes carried sticks to facilitate ointment application to the anus or genitals, where absorption occurred more rapidly. In order to avoid suspicion these may have been disguised as broomsticks or other apparently innocent items [22–24].

Modern day use of *Datura* is not infrequently reported in the USA, where it is commonly known as Jimson weed [2, 25, 26]. Abusers are typically adolescent males who seek hallucinogenic effects, usually by drinking an aqueous infusion of the plant material. The roots, seeds and leaves are all used but the seeds contain the most atropine. Occasionally the leaves are prepared as a 'reefer' and smoked. After oral administration, pharmacological effects begin within about an hour but may persist for up to 48 hours because antimuscarinic drugs inhibit the motility of the gastrointestinal tract and thereby reduce their own rate of absorption. The symptoms of antimuscarinic toxicity and intoxication are aptly described by the following lines:

Hot as a hare,	(hyperthermia)
Blind as a bat,	(dilated pupils)
Dry as a bone,	(dry mouth, reduced sweating)
Red as a beet,	(flushing)
Mad as a hatter.	(disorientation, incoherency, hallucination, agitation)

Other effects may include tachycardia, urinary retention, sedation, headache, nausea, vomiting, hyperreflexia, combative behaviour, seizures and coma. Several deaths have been reported. In 1994, the American Association of Poison Control Centers Toxic Exposure Surveillance System was notified of 318 cases of *Datura* toxicity [26].

PEYOTE CACTUS

The Peyote cactus, *Lophophora williamsii*, is found in the wild in Mexico and Texas. The heads of the cactus are eaten whole or are made into an infusion. The plant has been abused for at least 10 000 years by New World peoples such as the Aztecs. The psychoactive component mescaline is chemically related to the amphetamines and may produce hallucinations, out-of-the-body experiences and synaesthesia.

BETEL

The chewing of betel is widespread in India and Southeast Asia. Users prepare a 'quid' for chewing which contains three ingredients: betel 'nut' (seed of *Areca catechu*), betel leaf (leaf of *Piper betle*) and slaked lime. Chewing betel releases a red dye into the mouth.

Betel chewing produces a mild state of intoxication and euphoria. This effect is thought to be mediated via inhibition of GABA uptake in the brain. Arecoline is the main alkaloid constituent of *Areca catechu* but it is not itself psychoactive. However, chewing with lime results in arecoline hydrolysis to arecaidine and this product is a powerful inhibitor of GABA uptake [27]. The alkaline environment produced by the lime also facilitates absorption from the mouth.

Adverse effects from chewing betel include mouth ulcers, giddiness, abdominal pains and diarrhoea. Betel nut chewing has also been associated with acute attacks of asthma [28]. Oral cancer is known to be caused by the practise of betel chewing but is thought to be due to the slaked lime rather than the plant material itself [29]. Arecoline is a cholinergic agonist and is probably the cause of the gastrointestinal side effects of betel. It has also been reported to reduce the effectiveness of the antimuscarinic drug procyclidine in protecting against phenothiazine-induced extrapyramidal symptoms [30].

Withdrawal symptoms have been described in some users following discontinuation of chronic betel chewing. Lack of concentration, tiredness, anxiety, despondency and paranoia developed in two patients described by Wiesner after enforced cessation of a long-term habit [31].

GINSENG

A variety of plants are referred to as 'ginseng'. Usually the species taken is *Panax ginseng* (Korean, Chinese or Asian ginseng) which is known to produce CNS stimulation. In 1979, Siegel studied 133 ginseng users and described the 'ginseng abuse syndrome' [32]. This he characterised as 'hypertension together with nervousness, sleeplessness, skin eruptions and morning diarrhoea'. He noted that all sufferers also took caffeinated drinks but did not give details of the quantities consumed.

Some used up to 15 g of powdered ginseng root per day. Although most took ginseng orally, nine had experimented with intranasal administration and four had tried injection.

All users reported stimulation as an effect of ginseng and many described feelings of well-being or increased cognitive ability; euphoria was mentioned by 18 users. The CNS arousal produced by ginseng is probably effected by glycoside constituents which vary according to the species. Ginseng is also claimed to have a stimulant effect upon athletic performance but this has not been substantiated [33].

KAVA

Kava is a traditional beverage in the South Pacific Islands [34] and is derived from the macerated root and stem of a shrub, *Piper methysticum*. It has mild intoxicating and relaxant properties which are similar to those of alcohol. An extract has been found to be effective clinically as an anxiolytic [35]. The spread of chronic heavy kava abuse among the Aborigines of northern Australia in the 1980s caused much concern, not least because of the detrimental effects that it is known to have on general health (malnutrition, weight loss, hepatic/renal dysfunction, rash dyspnoea, etc.) [36–38].

EPHEDRA

There are about 40 species of *Ephedra*, amongst which are *E. sinica, E. equisetina, E. major* and *E. distachya*. All of them contain between 0.5 and 2 per cent alkaloids, of which up to 90 per cent are ephedrine and its isomers [39]. In traditional Chinese medicine, ephedra is known as Ma Huang and it is used as an anti-inflammatory. However, ephedrine is a sympathomimetic with properties similar to, although milder than, amphetamine and the plant has been the subject of abuse. In the USA it has been marketed as a legal alternative to illicit stimulants, under tradenames such as Herbal Ecstasy, Cloud 9 and Xphoria. In 1996, the plant was believed to have caused 15 deaths, leading at least one state to prohibit its sale [40]. Ephedrine-containing medicines have caused severe psychiatric disturbances such as psychosis and mania (see Chapter 12), and similar effects have been attributed to *Ephedra* ingestion [41, 42].

REFERENCES

1. Webb, E., Ashton, C.H., Kelly, P. and Kamali, F. (1996) Alcohol and drug use in UK university students. *Lancet*, **348**: 922–925.
2. Spoerke, D.G. and Hall, A.H. (1990) Plants and mushrooms of abuse. *Emerg. Med. Clin. N. Am.* **8**: 579–593.
3. Francis, J. and Murray, V.S.G. (1983) Review of enquiries made to the NPIS concerning *Psilocybe* mushroom ingestion 1978–1981. *Hum. Toxicol.* **2**: 349–352.

4. Peden, N.R., Bissett, A.F., Macaulay, K.E.C., Crooks, J. and Pelosi, A.J. (1981) Clinical toxicology of 'magic mushroom' ingestion. *Postgrad. Med. J.* **57**: 543–545.

5. Brenner, N., Frank, O.S. and Knight, E. (1993) Chronic nutmeg psychosis. *J. R. Soc. Med.* **86**: 179–180.

6. Panayotopoulos, D.J. and Chisholm, D.D. (1970) Hallucinogenic effect of nutmeg (letter). *Br. Med. J.* **i**: 754.

7. Faguet, R.A. and Rowland, K.F.(1978) 'Spice cabinet' intoxication. *Am. J. Psychiatr.* **135**: 860.

8. Lavy, G. (1987) Nutmeg intoxication in pregnancy. A case report. *J. Reprod. Med.* **32**: 63–64.

9. Kalix, P. (1988) Khat: a plant with amphetamine effects. *J. Subst. Abuse Treat.* **5**: 163–169.

10. Kalix P. (1987) Khat: scientific knowledge and policy issues. *Br. J. Addict.* **82**: 47–53.

11. Pantelis, C., Hindler, C.G. and Taylor, J.C. (1989) Use and abuse of khat (*Catha edulis*): a review of the distribution, pharmacology, side effects and a description of psychosis attributed to khat chewing. *J. Psychol. Med.* **19**: 657–688.

12. Critchlow, S. and Seifert, R. (1987) Khat-induced paranoid psychosis. *Br. J. Psychiatr.* **150**: 247–249.

13. Jager, A.D. and Siveling, L. (1994) Natural history of khat psychosis. *Aust. N. Z. J. Psychiatr.* **28**: 331–332.

14. Giannini, A.J., Miller, N.S. and Turner, C.E. (1992) Treatment of khat addiction. *J. Subst. Abuse Treat.* **9**: 379–382.

15. Soufi, H.E., Kameswaran, M. and Malatani, T. (1991) Khat and oral cancer. *J. Laryngol. Otol.* **105**: 643–645.

16. El-Shoura, S.M., Abdel Aziz, M., Ali, M.E. *et al..* (1995) Deleterious effects of khat addiction on semen parameters and sperm ultrastructure. *Hum. Reprod.* **10**: 2295–2300.

17. Goudie, A.J. (1987). Importing khat, legal but dangerous (letter). *Lancet*, **330**: 1340–1341.

18. Capper K.R. (1968) Lysergic acid derivatives in morning glory seeds, in *The Pharmacological and Epidemiological Aspects of Adolescent Drug Dependence*, (ed. C.W.M. Wilson), Pergamon Press, New York, pp. 75–81.

19. Briggs, C. (1992) Guarana. *Can. Pharm. J.* May, 222–224.

20. Houghton, P. (1995) Guarana. *Pharm. J.* **254**: 435–436.

21. Aktuell (1993) Guarana – der 'neue' Muntermacher. *Dtsch. Apotheker Zeit.* **133**: 218.

22. Richardson, P.M. (1988) *Encyclopedia of Psychoactive Drugs: Flowering Plants – Magic in Bloom* (British edition), Burke Publishing Co., London.

23. Rudgley, R. (1993) *The Alchemy of Culture: Intoxicants in Society*, British Museum Press, London, pp. 90–99.

24. Harner, M.J. (ed) (1973) The role of hallucinogenic plants in European

witchcraft, in *Hallucinogens and Shamaninsm*, Oxford University Press, London, pp. 126–150.

25. Shervette, R.E., Schydlower, M., Lampe, R.M. and Fearnow, R.G. (1979) Jimson 'loco' weed abuse in adolescents. *Pediatrics*, **63**: 520–523.

26. From the CDC (1995) Jimson weed poisoning – Texas, New York and California 1994. *J. Am. Med. Assoc.* **273**: 532–533.

27. Johnston, G.A.R., Kroggaard-Larsen, P. and Stephenson, A. (1975) Betel nut constituents as inhibitors of gamma-aminobutyric acid uptake. *Nature*, **258**: 627-628.

28. Taylor, R.F.H., Al-Jarad, N., John, L.M.E., Conroy, D.M. and Barnes, N.C. (1992) Betel-nut chewing and asthma. *Lancet*, **339**: 1134–1136.

29. Thomas, S.J. and Maclennan, R. (1992) Slaked lime and betel nut cancer in Papua New Guinea. *Lancet*, **340**: 577–578.

30. Deahl, M.P. (1987) Psychostimulant properties of betel nuts (letter). *Br. Med. J.* **294**: 849.

31. Wiesner, D.M. (1987) Betel nut withdrawal. *Med. J. Aust.* **146**: 453.

32. Siegel R.K. (1979) Ginseng abuse syndrome – problems with the panacea. *J. Am. Med. Assoc.* **241**: 1614–1615.

33. Bahrke, M.S. and Morgan, W.P. (1994) Evaluation of the ergogenic properties of ginseng. *Sports Med.* **18**: 229–248.

34. Singh, Y.N. (1992) Kava: an overview. *J. Ethnopharmacol.* **37**: 13–45.

35. Kinzler, E., Kromer, J. and Lehmann, E. (1991) Wirksamkeit eines Kava-Spezial-Extraktes bei Patienten mit Angst-, Spannungs-, und Erregungszustanden nich-psychotischer Genese. *Arzneim. Forsch.* **41**: 584.

36. Cawte, J. (1988) Macabre effects of a 'cult' for kava. *Med. J. Aust.* **148**: 545–546.

37. Mathews, J.D., Riley, M.D., Fejo, L. *et al.* (1988) Effects of the heavy usage of kava on physical health: summary of a pilot survey in an Aboriginal community. *Med. J. Aust.* **148**: 548–555.

38. Editorial (1988) Kava. *Lancet*, **332**: 258–259.

39. Trease, G.E. and Evans, W.C. (1983) *Pharmacognosy*, Bailiere Tindall, London, pp. 572–573.

40. Josefson, D. (1996) Herbal stimulant causes US deaths. *Br. Med. J.* **312**: 1441.

41. Capwell, R.R. (1995) Ephedrine induced mania from a herbal diet supplement. *Am. J. Psychiatr.* **152**: 647.

42. Doyle, H. and Kargin, M. (1996) Herbal stimulant containing ephedrine has also caused psychosis. *Br. Med. J.* **313**: 756.

17

Alkyl nitrites

Poppers make you feel really heady when you're dancing but you have to keep sniffing it every few minutes because it doesn't last long. Sometimes it makes you feel a bit dizzy.

Comment from user, 1996.

HISTORY

Three alkyl nitrites are commonly abused: amyl nitrite, butyl nitrite and isobutyl nitrite. Amyl nitrite was used from 1867 until the earlier part of this century as a treatment for angina attacks. It was supplied in small glass 'capsules' (or vitrellae) which were broken open during an attack of angina and the contents inhaled. The nitrites are essentially vasodilators, being converted to the endogenous mediator nitric oxide *in vivo*.

The popping sound made when vitrellae were broken has given rise to the most popular street name for nitrites: 'poppers'. The name has persisted despite the fact that this particular preparation has not been available at street level for many years. Amyl nitrite is currently a 'pharmacy' medicine and so supplies in any form are limited. The Medicines Control Agency has proposed that it should be rendered a prescription only drug [1]. This proposal would not apply to other alkyl nitrites. Butyl and isobutyl nitrites are used far more frequently than amyl nitrite at street level because until recently the sale of these nitrites was not thought to have been covered by the Medicines Act. As a consequence, they could be sold freely anywhere without a prescription, usually under the guise of 'room odourisers' to avoid claiming medicinal or intoxicating properties. However, a test case was recently brought by the Royal Pharmaceutical Society in which it was ruled that the sale of butyl and isobutyl nitrites to the public was illegal in the UK because they were medicinal products [2]. It remains to be seen whether this decision can or will be enforced. Abuse, possession or supply of nitrites does not contravene the Misuse of Drugs Act in the UK but in the USA amyl, butyl and isobutyl nitrites are illegal substances. This has led to the limited, and legal, abuse of propyl nitrites in some states.

ADMINISTRATION

The alkyl nitrites are volatile yellowish clear liquids which have a distinctive smell, often likened to 'old socks'. The liquid is irritant and may burn the skin if spilled. It is also inflammable and so care should be taken to avoid contact with fire (e.g. lighted cigarettes).

Nitrites are inhaled, usually directly from a small bottle. Some examples are shown in Figure 17.1. Rapid deep inhalation produces a sudden intense 'buzz' of excitement. This is often referred to by users as a 'rush' or 'high'. The effects only last a few minutes. Users typically repeat the inhalation at regular intervals to maintain the effect.

Butyl nitrite is available from most sex shops and is also sold at night clubs and some pubs and bars. It is usually supplied in small thumb-sized bottles which cost around £5 each. Nitrites are usually known on the street as 'poppers'. Brand names of nitrite products include Rush, Stud, TNT, Locker Room and Liquid Gold. The extent of use in the UK is not known, although a survey of 3075 second-year university

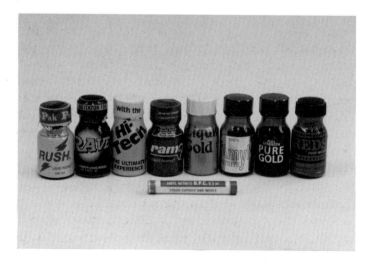

Figure 17.1 A selection of 'poppers' available in the UK.

students from around the country in 1996 revealed that 15 per cent had used alkyl nitrites at least once [3]. Only 0.8 per cent of the total surveyed were regular users (at least once every week).

EFFECTS SOUGHT

Those who abuse nitrites may do so simply to experience the 'rush'. Others may use nitrites to loosen inhibition on the dance floor at night-clubs, often in association with other drugs such as ecstasy. Some believe that nitrites may enhance the effects of ecstasy. Certain users believe that nitrites can heighten creativity or the perception of music.

Others use nitrites during intercourse because they claim that nitrites seem to enhance sexual experience and prolong orgasm. Homosexual men may use the drug to relax the anal muscles during anal intercourse.

ADVERSE EFFECTS

Not all users find the euphoria produced by nitrites pleasant [4–9]. In a survey conducted in Virginia, 32 out of a total of 73 who had used the drug found the experience unpleasant [4].

The following effects are common after inhalation of nitrites:

- light-headedness, dizziness;
- flushing of the face, feeling hot, tachycardia, palpitations;
- headache;
- inflammation or a 'burning' sensation around the mouth and nose.

Less common effects include blurred vision, weakness, cold sweats, fainting and nausea. A rash, dermatitis, wheezing or inflammation of the eye can also occur. Methaemoglobinaemia, psychosis-like episodes and sudden death have been reported but these are extremely rare. Methaemoglobinaemia can be fatal but usually only in those who have ingested large quantities, rather than inhaled. The symptoms are those of acute anaemia due to the decreased oxygen-carrying capacity of the blood. In most cases the effect is reversible but this particular toxic effect can persist for an hour or so, i.e. considerably longer than the intoxicating effects. Nitrites may theoretically worsen glaucoma but the short duration of action makes a clinically significant effect unlikely. Nitrites should be avoided by those with hypotension or heart failure. It has been suggested that nitrites could cause Kaposi's sarcoma in patients with AIDS [5, 6] but the evidence is circumstantial. However, nitrites do have immunosuppressive effects and so are best avoided by those with compromised immunity [6, 8, 9] (see Chapter 19). These effects upon immunity can persist for a few days after exposure but are reversible. In addition, nitrites may be metabolised to nitrosamines *in vivo* which could be carcinogenic.

There are no proven long-term side effects of nitrites. Nitrites do not produce dependence and tolerance is most unlikely due to the very short half-lives of the drugs involved.

REFERENCES

1.   Anon. (1996) Latest MCA proposals include POM control for amyl nitrite. *Pharm. J.* **257**: 174.
2.   Anon. (1996) Society wins 'poppers' case at a price. *Pharm. J.* **256**: 883.
3.   Webb, E., Ashton, C.H., Kelly, P. and Kamali, F. (1996) Alcohol and drug use in UK university students. *Lancet*, **348**: 922–925.
4.   Schwartz, R.H. and Peary, P. (1986) Abuse of isobutyl nitrite inhalation (Rush) by adolescents. *Clin. Pediatr.* **25**: 308–310.
5.   Mathur-Wagh, U., Mildvan, D. and Senie, R.T. (1985) Follow-up at four and a half years on homosexual men with generalized lymphadenopathy (letter). *N. Engl. J. Med.* **313**: 1542–1543.
6.   Lange, W.R. and Fralich, J. (1989) Nitrite inhalants: promising and discouraging news (editorial). *Br. J. Addict.* **84**: 121–123.
7.   Sigell, L.T., Kapp, F.T., Fusaro, G.A., Nelson, E.D. and Falck, R.S. (1978) Popping and snorting volatile nitrites: a current fad for getting high. *Am. J. Psychiatr.* **135**: 1216–1218.
8.   Lockwood, B. (1996) Poppers: volatile nitrite inhalants. *Pharm. J.* **257**: 154–155.
9.   Anon. (1994) *Drug Notes: Poppers.* Institute for the Study of Drug Dependence, London, pp.1–6.

18

Smart drugs

It is never wise to try to appear to be more clever than you are. It is sometimes wise to appear slightly less so.
William Whitelaw, 'Sayings of the Year',
The Observer, 1975.

Smart drugs are also known as 'cognition enhancers'; a subclass of compounds are referred to as 'nootropics' (especially the pyrrolidone derivatives, see Table 18.1). Nootropics are claimed to improve or activate the natural processes of cognition without the sedative, stimulant or other adverse effects of traditional psychotropic drugs. The precise differences between nootropics and other cognition enhancers are not very well defined by proponents. Smart drugs are generally asserted to increase learning ability in healthy people and to induce keener perception, improved memory, sharpened concentration and, even, greater intelligence. Most of those involved in taking smart drugs are ambitious, healthy young people who want to increase their mental powers. Smart drugs have been the subject of discussion in many popular magazines and newspapers [1–4].

Parallels have been drawn between the use of smart drugs to enhance mental performance and the use of anabolic steroids to enhance physical performance [5]. Both groups of drugs may be taken to enhance social prowess, rather than to achieve euphoria or psychoactive effects. A questionnaire study of 193 students at the University of Virginia in 1994 revealed that although 26 per cent of the population were familiar with the term 'smart drugs' only 2.1 per cent reported using one [5].

ABUSE LIABILITY

It is easy to see why users might object to smart drugs being referred to as drugs of abuse. And perhaps this is an unfair description. Unlike most classical drugs of abuse, smart drugs are said to facilitate natural mental processes rather than to produce aberrant or novel psychoactive effects. They also do not cause dependence or withdrawal reactions. However, smart drugs do share some characteristics with more conventionally defined drugs of abuse.

- They are pharmacologically active substances which are not taken for a medical condition.
- The potential for side effects is not appreciated by users.
- The long-term mental consequences of administration are not known in most cases.
- There could be important social or financial consequences arising from widespead use of these substances whether they produce the desired effects or not.
- The pharmaceutical purity, quality and identity of many of the substances purchased is not regulated and is open to question.

The last points might equally apply to many 'alternative medicine' or herbal products, consequently smart drugs might superficially appear no different from any other health food 'fad'. However, there are important differences other than those given above. First, a large number of products is involved: over 140 are currently being used or investigated. Table 18.1 lists some of these. Secondly, there are great financial pressures behind smart drugs. In the USA, the domestic market for such products has been estimated at over $40m for 1994. A third difference is that several large pharmaceutical companies have an interest in the marketing of cognition-enhancing drugs. A final important point is that some advocates of smart drugs encourage the unsupervised use of certain prescription only medicines as cognition enhancers. This clearly could be dangerous. Table 18.1 also includes some of these.

AVAILABILITY

None of the smart drugs are controlled by drug misuse legislation and so possession of these substances is not illegal. In the USA, and to a lesser extent in the UK, a range of products is sold in health food outlets and bars with names such as 'memory booster' and 'memory fuel'. These are often merely combinations of simple nutrients. Most of the more pharmacologically active smart drugs are only available by mail order.

Table 18.1   Examples of smart drugs

Pyrrolidone derivatives
- Piracetam, pramiracetam, oxiracetam, aniracetam, nebracetam

Nutrients
- Vitamin B_{12} (and other B group vitamins)
- Vitamin E
- Dimethylaminoethanol (DMAE or deanol)
- Pyroglutamate, phenylalanine

Acetylcholine 'enhancers'
- Choline, lecithin, inositol
- Acetyl-L-carnitine (ST200)

Plant-derived products
- Ginseng
- Ginkgo biloba
- Vincamine, vinpocetine (Periwinkle plant)
- Co-dergocrine mesylate (Hydergine, ergot derived)

UK prescription only medicines
- Selegiline, levodopa, bromocriptine
- Phenytoin
- Nimodipine
- Vasopressin
- Propranolol
- Procaine
- Meclofenoxate (centrophenoxine)

A legal loophole in the UK allows members of the public to purchase prescription only medicines from overseas suppliers if these are for personal use. This means that the public can import drugs such as bromocriptine, propranolol and vasopressin for use without medical supervision. It is, however, illegal for those importing these prescription only drugs to supply them to a third party within the UK.

Sometimes single drugs are administered; other users take cocktails or mixtures of various products which have alleged synergism. All are taken orally, with the notable exception of vasopressin which is usually inhaled nasally. Proponents claim that vasopressin has a rapid onset via this route and can thus be taken when required as a quick 'cognitive top-up' for mentally demanding situations.

DEVELOPMENT OF SMART DRUGS

At first sight, the use of a drug to improve cognition seems feasible. After all, some substances are known to cause memory impairment (e.g. antimuscarinic agents, alcohol and the benzodiazepines). However, closer examination reveals a more complex situation.

Information about smart drugs has largely arisen from the pharmacological manipulation of learning behaviour in animals and the treatment of dementia/cognitive decline in aged humans and animals. A number of the drugs listed in Table 18.1 are known to improve rodent learning and memory in maze-deciphering and similar experiments; furthermore, some drugs seem to have 'antiamnesic' effects for both reward behaviour and situations where animals learn to avoid a noxious stimulus.

In addition, over the past two decades many of the substances listed have been studied as possible treatments for the cognitive impairment that accompanies certain forms of dementia, such as Alzheimer's disease. It is widely accepted that cholinergic nerves have an important role in learning behaviour. It is also known that central production of acetylcholine declines with age and this loss may be particularly marked in those with Alzheimer's disease. Consequently, many of the drugs investigated initially were agents that sought to boost cholinergic activity of the brain by acting as precursors to acetylcholine synthesis or by inhibiting the breakdown of this neurotransmitter. Other approaches have sought to increase blood flow to the central nervous system by vasodilation, to influence brain metabolism or to increase the activity of other neurotransmitter systems. Often the mode of action is unclear.

Despite the extensive investigation, the simple fact is that no drug currently available will substantially reverse the cognitive changes which occur in senile dementia enabling the affected individual to lead a normal life. Several of the drugs in Table 18.1 have been tested in demented patients but, despite promising theories, clinical results have proved disappointing. Certain drugs may have minor impact on particular tests of cognition but none of them significantly improves the patient's quality of life in a meaningful way. Some may slow down the deterioration but none of them substantially reverses the process.

CLAIMS MADE FOR SMART DRUGS

The supporters of smart drugs can produce an impressive-sounding array of scientific papers to back up their claims. Unfortunately, none of these studies has involved the target population for smart drugs, i.e. non-demented, healthy and (mostly) young people who want to increase their 'brain power'.

A high proportion of the research quoted involves the animal studies which have already been alluded to. While much of this work does show that, for example, a particular smart drug will help a rat remember which way to run around a maze, one cannot help but wonder: is this relevant to humans? What does a drug-induced change in animal behaviour really mean in this situation? There is an assumption that changes in animal behaviour in the laboratory can be extrapolated to the human condition. Yet the human brain is larger and more complex, and human learning or memory can be influenced by a vast array of environmental, personal and social pressures to which laboratory animals cannot be subject. Supporters also assume that the basic neurobiochemical processes of learning/memory are the same in all mammals, which is by no means proven. In addition, animal tests can be difficult to standardise, poorly reproducible and subject to many variables. Can changes in laboratory animals be seriously related to something as intangible as human intellect and memory?

Other evidence cited to support the use of smart drugs in healthy people includes studies of demented patients, as discussed above. These experiments have produced disappointing, often conflicting, results. Where improvement does occur this is frequently limited to a marginal change in a small number of the mental tests and psychometric assessments which were performed. It is clearly unreasonable to extrapolate the minimal improvements seen in tests of demented patients to cognition enhancement in healthy unaffected people. The brain of the demented subject is functioning below the normal standard and would not be expected to respond to drug treatment in the same way as a healthy brain. It is not unreasonable to believe that a drug might improve cognition if there is a disease-related cause for decline. But to imply that these drugs should work in an otherwise healthy brain suggests that the central nervous system normally functions at suboptimal capacity. This does not seem logical.

Much of the research quoted to support smart drugs has been published in obscure journals where the quality of refereeing might be open to question. Sometimes the studies are poorly designed; using small numbers of participants, giving vague unquantified results and sometimes even involving administration of smart drugs by unrepresentative routes which the general population would not use (e.g. intravenous, intracerebral). Statistical analysis is often dubious. The lack of a consistent mode of action for the different smart drugs – even those with a similar chemical structure – also tends to promote disbelief.

A further complication is that some drugs which are claimed to enhance cognition may actually be removing barriers to memory or intellect rather than boosting mental processes directly. For example, several of the smart drugs have anxiolytic, stimulant, antidepressant, anti-Parkinsonian or psychotropic effects which may help overcome obstacles to cognition, rather than improving 'brain power' *per se.*

The final evidence that smart drug advocates produce is the testimonials of users. Where these are genuine, there is no evidence that they are anything other than a placebo response. It is known that the placebo effect can be particularly marked when psychological/psychiatric conditions are treated [6]. The goal of treatment in these cases is often a change in behaviour or mentation rather than an easily measured physical change. Placebo-controlled, blind trials need to be conducted in healthy young volunteers before the scientific community can evaluate any potential benefits of cognition-enhancing drugs in the healthy population.

MODES OF ACTION

In retrospect, it seems naïve that the early investigators of dementia could have hoped that simply increasing brain levels of acetylcholine would be sufficient to dramatically improve a behaviour as complex as memory and learning. However, a variety of cholinergic enhancers are still used as smart drugs. Choline and lecithin, for example, are converted into acetylcholine by metabolism. Tacrine and velnacrine inhibit the breakdown of acetylcholine but although widely investigated for the treatment of dementia they do not appear to have been used commonly as smart drugs. The pyrrolidone derivatives may also enhance the effectiveness of central cholinergic systems, although this group of drugs probably has additional important actions via aldosterone and glucose metabolism. Their structural similarity to GABA (gamma-aminobutyric acid) might also be relevant.

Certain cognitive enhancers may increase cerebral blood flow by vasodilation (e.g. vinpocetine), facilitate calcium passage across neurones (e.g. nimodipine) or affect neural growth/repair. Drugs that act via specific neurotransmitters are also claimed to have cognition-enhancing effects, e.g. ondansetron (acting on 5-hydroxytryptamine, 5HT) and levodopa (dopamine). A range of other neurotransmitter systems may also be implicated, including GABA, glutamate, endogenous opioids and beta-adrenoceptors.

Some drugs (e.g. acetyl-L-carnitine) seem able to reduce lipofuscin deposits in the brains of experimental animals. This substance accumulates in the brain with age and may be a cause of neuronal damage. Certain drugs have free radical scavenging properties (e.g. dimethylaminoethanol) or are antioxidants (e.g. vitamin E). As may be expected, most of the smart drugs have a multiplicity of pharmacological actions.

FUTURE USE OF SMART DRUGS

Supporters of smart drugs and associated pharmacotherapy have attempted to link use of these substances with the profitable anti-ageing industry. The condition of age-associated memory impairment (AAMI) has been proposed and supported by certain pharmaceutical companies active in the investigation of cognition. This has occurred largely in response to the realisation that the drug regulatory authorities are unlikely to allow cognitive enhancers to be marketed without definite treatment goals. And this means identifying a condition to be treated in the first place!

The objective of pharmaceutical manufacturers is presumably to launch drugs which may treat or prevent the normal (non-dementia) deterioration in memory that naturally accompanies advancing age. But is this a condition which should be treated? Is attempting to change this natural age-related effect the same as, say, fitting a hearing aid or treating maturity-onset diabetes? Those selling smart drugs pluck on a notable chord in many people: the desire to be a 'better' person: to perform well in examinations, to obtain a better job, to be more educated. Would any of these objectives be as worthwhile if they were achieved with minimum effort and a tablet, rather than with determined hard work?

If smart drugs are proven to boost memory and intelligence in healthy people, the majority of the population will presumably want to take them from childhood upwards. If this treatment is not available on the National Health Service, will only the rich be able to afford these 'elitist' drugs? Must one take the drug for life to continue to experience the beneficial effects? If so, will long-term treatment affect the neurobiochemical make-up of the brain in other perhaps undesirable ways?

Alternatively, might smart drugs offer all of us the chance to achieve more, to release an untapped intellectual resource, perhaps to live to old age without fear of dementia?

Fortunately, we do not have to consider answers to any of these questions yet because there is no reliable evidence that any of the existing smart drugs increases cognition in healthy people in a useful way.

REFERENCES

1. Heley, M. (1991) High time to get smart. *Weekend Guardian*, 8–9 June, pp. 14–15.
2. Concar, D. and Coghlan, A. (1993) Is there money in lost memories? *New Scientist*, 17 April, pp. 20–22.
3. Rose, S. (1993) No way to treat the mind. *New Scientist*, 17 April, pp. 23–26.
4. Anon. (1993) Smart drugs. *Which? Way to Health*, February, pp. 22–25.
5. Canterbury, R.J. and Lloyd, E. (1994) Smart drugs: implications of student use. *J. Primary Prev.* **14**: 197–207.
6. Laporte, J.-R. and Figueras, A. (1994) Placebo effects in psychiatry. *Lancet*, **344**: 1206–1209.

FURTHER READING

1. Dean, W. and Morgenthaler, J. (1990) *Smart Drugs and Nutrients – How to Improve Your Memory and Increase Your Intelligence Using the Latest Discoveries in Neuroscience.* B & J Publications, Santa Cruz.

19

Drug abuse and concurrent illness

Illness is in part what the world has done to a victim but in a larger part is what the victim has done with his world, and with himself.

Karl Menninger, quoted in 'Illness as Metaphor' by Susan Sontag.

From time to time the healthcare professional will encounter an individual with a medical condition who abuses drugs. Although not condoning the taking of these substances, it is desirable that those in a position to advise are able to provide information on whether the drug is liable to exacerbate the condition. The sections below provide brief details which may be helpful in advising those with some of the more common medical conditions. The information given should be used as a guide only. The data available are sparse in most cases and while it is hoped that the details in this chapter will be useful, every patient's particular circumstances will differ and one should be cautious about extrapolating limited information to all situations in which it could be applicable.

It is difficult to find data on the advisability of drug abuse in those suffering from concomitant medical conditions. The data given here are based upon details of side effects that have been reported in the medical literature and knowledge of drug handling by the body. This information is incomplete because none of the drugs of abuse have been subject to large-scale clinical trials at the doses abused. This is the main mechanism by which side effect profiles of therapeutic drugs are determined. This being the case, most of the data on adverse effects from street drugs are derived from small-scale studies, case reports, surveys and anecdotal evidence. Causality can also be difficult to ascertain because many users employ a variety of drugs simultaneously. Many drug abusers have a poor quality of life due to bad living conditions and/or inadequate nutrition; this may make them more susceptible to various diseases.

This book considers a large number of individual drugs of abuse. For the purpose of this chapter the drugs considered will be those which are most commonly encountered: opioids, LSD, amphetamines and ecstasy, cannabis, cocaine, volatile substances, alkyl nitrites, benzodiazepines, anabolic steroids, caffeine, alcohol, tobacco and antimuscarinics.

ASTHMA

The drugs which are inhaled or smoked are most likely to cause respiratory symptoms. When taken in this way, cocaine can cause cough [1], bronchospasm [2], wheezing [3] and even status asthmaticus [4]. It has also been associated with a hypersensitivity reaction which is characterised by breathlessness, cough and pyrexia [5]. Hypersensitivity to any drug of abuse can manifest as bronchospasm – this reaction has even been associated with alcohol [6] – but in many cases it can be difficult to determine whether the individual is hypersensitive to the drug of abuse or to any adulterants or additives present.

When smoked, cannabis and tobacco impair gaseous exchange, deposit tar in the lungs and can cause bronchitis. The inhalation of smoke particles can trigger an asthmatic attack either in the smoker or in those subject to passive smoking. Regular smoking of cannabis or tobacco usually results in a markedly increased metabolism of theophylline [7], a drug widely used in the treatment of asthma. Increased metabolism of theophylline gives rise to decreased duration of action and reduced concentrations of the drug in plasma.

Overdose of intravenous opioids can cause bronchospasm, respiratory arrest and pulmonary oedema. However in the absence of overdose, heroin is occasionally reported to cause bronchospasm when injected [8] or vaporised [9] although the role of adulterants in eliciting this response is unclear. Repeated injection of any street drug can cause pulmonary talcosis due to the presence of insoluble excipients or adulterants in the liquid injected. These can accumulate in small blood vessels in the lung and cause respiratory distress.

Theoretically, large doses of benzodiazepines can cause respiratory depression but in practice even large doses fail to have a significant effect upon respiration unless the individual has moderate to severe pre-existing respiratory impairment.

DIABETES

Alcohol can cause hypoglycaemia by a variety of mechanisms. It may be delayed by up to 36 hours but it usually only occurs after acute ingestion of large quantities of alcohol [10]. Alcohol may also potentiate the effects of insulin or oral hypoglycaemic drugs. Chronic heavy drinking is commonly associated with hyperglycaemia, glucose intolerance or frank diabetes [11]. Drinking within nationally recommended limits is not likely to have adverse effects on glycaemic control. Cannabis has been reported to cause a slight increase in blood glucose but this is not clinically relevant unless large doses are taken regularly and even then the reaction is very rare [12]. Insulin-dependent diabetics that smoke require up to 30 per cent more insulin than non-smokers [13]. This means that diabetics that start or stop smoking are likely to have to adjust their insulin requirement. Conversely, diabetics given certain anabolic steroids seem to require much less insulin [14]. It is not clear whether this effect can occur with all steroids; it has been reported for nandrolone, stanozolol, methandienone and testosterone.

Certain drugs might be expected to affect glycaemic control in other ways. The stimulant drugs amphetamine, ecstasy and cocaine can all cause loss of appetite, which could lead to hypoglycaemia in diabetics who do not reduce doses of insulin or sulphonylurea once food intake declines. Cannabis, on the other hand, can increase appetite. The balance of food intake and dose of hypoglycaemic drug can also be disrupted by vomiting, which is a recognised side effect of most drugs of abuse except LSD, caffeine, benzodiazepines, nitrites and anabolic steroids. The stimulant drugs and anabolic steroids also increase stamina which could result in hypoglycaemia due to overactivity.

The apathy and poor motivation engendered in some individuals by chronic drug dependence may mitigate against adequate control of blood glucose. Non-compliance with diet, failure to administer medication correctly or inadequate monitoring could result from this. Intoxication may prevent a diabetic recognising and/or dealing with a hypoglycaemic episode. The hypoglycaemic episode can also resemble intoxication, so bystanders may not seek medical attention.

In one study, 26 out of 79 adolescent diabetics stated that alcohol or drugs had altered their diabetic control but no further details were provided [15].

EPILEPSY

Very little research has been performed into the effects of drug abuse on epilepsy. However, it is known that certain drugs can cause convulsions and so, as with therapeutic drugs that have proconvulsant properties, one would assume that epileptics would be more prone to this effect and should preferably avoid these drugs.

Of all the illicit drugs, cocaine probably has the strongest association with drug-induced convulsions. Alldredge *et al.* described 23 cases in San Francisco where cocaine was the sole drug taken [16]; seizures were reported following administration of cocaine by any route. Other reviews have similarly established a link between cocaine abuse and convulsions [17, 18]. The reaction is also a well-known symptom of cocaine overdose [19]. However, one study of 308 patients presenting to a casualty department in New York with seizures failed to identify cocaine as a risk factor despite it being commonly abused by patients and by controls [20].

Amphetamine has been linked to drug-induced fits but the link is less well established. Eight suspected cases in non-epileptics were reported in one US study [16]. Ecstasy would be expected to be capable of causing convulsions because it is an amphetamine derivative. Both ecstasy and amphetamine can cause fits as part of the sequelae of drug-induced hyperpyrexia or hyponatraemia (see Chapter 6) but, outside these scenarios, ecstasy-induced fits have not been described in the medical literature. Phencyclidine is known to cause seizures after both normal street-level doses and after overdose.

Fits may occur as a sign of heavy alcohol abuse or, more commonly, as a result of alcohol withdrawal. Chronic, regular, high intake of alcohol also accelerates the metabolism of the commonly used anticonvulsant phenytoin. Benzodiazepine withdrawal can cause convulsions but this is not common and tends to occur mainly with the shorter acting forms such as lorazepam. Heroin abuse is associated with fitting [16, 20], as are other opioids when used in high dose therapeutically. However, this effect of therapeutic opioids has been attributed to accumulation of preservatives [21] or to the misdiagnosis of intense opioid-induced muscular rigidity [22]. Opioid withdrawal is not associated with convulsions in adults but seizures have been occasionally described in neonates undergoing withdrawal due to *in utero* exposure. Overdose with dextropropoxyphene or pethidine is particularly linked to drug-induced fitting. Use of pethidine or pethidine analogues in patients with renal failure has also been associated with convulsions due to accumulation of a neurotoxic metabolite, norpethidine.

Caffeine can probably cause fits, as can the closely related theophylline but only after extremely large doses which would be unattainable by all but the most fanatical imbiber. Cannabis has been described as a cause of seizures in only one published case report [23]. However, Feeney reported 13 epileptics who used cannabis; one stated that the drug decreased his seizure frequency, another said that cannabis caused his seizures [24] and the remainder felt that cannabis had no effect. Most studies suggest that if cannabis has any effect at all on epilepsy, it should protect against convulsions [20, 25, 26]. Some of the constituent cannabinoids have been used for this purpose therapeutically [27].

Benzodiazepines would be expected to protect against convulsions. However, this group of drugs can have an unpredictable effect upon plasma phenytoin levels. Reports of increased, decreased and unaltered levels have been described [28].

The following drugs have not been reported to cause convulsions: LSD, nitrites, volatile substances, benzodiazepines (non-withdrawal), tobacco, antimuscarinics and anabolic steroids.

HEPATIC FAILURE

In individuals with impaired hepatic function, it is important to consider the potential toxic effects of drugs of abuse upon the liver as well as the effect of decreased hepatic function upon the clearance of these drugs.

Hepatotoxicity

In terms of the potential to cause hepatotoxicity, the drugs of abuse can be divided into three groups as follows:

Non-hepatotoxic

There is no evidence, or insufficient evidence, for certain drugs of abuse causing liver damage. These drugs are cannabis, LSD, caffeine, tobacco, alkyl nitrites and antimuscarinics.

Weak link to hepatotoxicity

For the drugs in this category, the evidence for hepatotoxicity comes from a small number of case reports, and/or the reaction is very rare, and/or the validity of reported observations have been questioned. The drugs in this category are the following:

Benzodiazepines   Cholestasis and hepatocellular injury have been attributed to this group of drugs. In reviewing the literature, the number of cases is small compared to the very wide usage of benzodiazepines and in many cases patients are reported as taking other drugs known to be hepatotoxic at the same time [29].

Amphetamine   The number of reported cases is small. More cases have been described with the related drug ecstasy (see below).

Volatile substances   Hepatic damage is a rare complication of trichloroethylene abuse [30] and of toluene abuse [31, 32].

Cocaine   Cocaine is hepatotoxic in mice [33]. In humans, minor elevation of various liver enzyme levels is quite common in cocaine abusers [34]. Hepatic necrosis has also been reported, including fatal cases [35, 36] but, in a detailed review, Farrell concluded that there was insufficient evidence for cocaine being directly hepatotoxic in humans. In all published cases, human liver damage could be attributed to hepatic ischaemia as all patients involved were suffering from shock, hypotension, hyperpyrexia, rhabdomyolysis or renal failure [33]. By contrast, *in vitro* experiments with human liver cells suggest that cocaine can be directly cytotoxic and that alcohol could potentiate the hepatoxicity of cocaine [37] under the test conditions. However, in turn, these results were not confirmed in a large study of human alcoholics that abused cocaine [38].

Opioids   Reports of opioid-induced hepatic failure are extremely rare. Liver biopsies have shown that those who inject heroin may have sinusoidal dilatation, and sinusoidal and hepatic vein inflammation. In ex-abusers this inflammation is largely replaced by fibrosis [39]. However, the functional significance of these changes is unclear. Studies using cultured human hepatocytes have suggested that alcohol may potentiate the cytotoxic actions of heroin and methadone [40].

Well-established hepatotoxicity

It has been clearly documented that alcohol, anabolic steroids and ecstasy can cause liver damage.

Alcohol is associated with a range of liver disorders [41]. Fatty liver can occur to some degree in anyone who drinks a large amount of alcohol, even when this is episodic. It appears to be a dose-related phenomenon and is usually completely reversible when alcohol intake ceases. Acute alcoholic hepatitis occurs as a result of chronic high alcohol intake and involves an inflammatory reaction within the liver, often accompanied by fatty change and jaundice. It is probably reversible if the individual survives and stops drinking but may be a precursor to alcoholic cirrhosis. Cirrhosis itself occurs subsequent to many years of heavy drinking and may progress to hepatocellular carcinoma.

Anabolic steroids are known to cause cholestatic jaundice, which is usually reversible but can rarely progress to peliosis hepatis. Adenoma and hepatocellular carcinoma are also potential adverse effects [42]. Ecstasy has been reported to cause acute hepatitis accompanied by jaundice [43–45].

Drug accumulation in hepatic failure

All of the drugs of abuse considered in this chapter except three are largely eliminated via the liver, so hepatic failure may allow any of them to accumulate to a greater or lesser extent. The exceptions are :

- Ecstasy. This is mainly eliminated renally (about two-thirds), so hepatic failure may make little difference to clearance.
- Volatile substances. Most volatile substances are excreted via the lungs, so that even in severe liver failure they will be cleared normally. Toluene is an exception since it is partly liver metabolised.
- Cocaine. This is largely metabolised by pseudocholinesterases which are concentrated in the liver but also found elsewhere throughout the body. Liver failure may therefore not seriously impair cocaine clearance.

HYPERTENSION

Cocaine and amphetamines are known to increase blood pressure and should be avoided by those with hypertension. Anabolic steroids may have a similar effect because they encourage fluid retention. Chronic moderate to high alcohol intake also raises blood pressure. In addition, alcohol can exacerbate the postural hypotensive response to many anti-hypertensives. The other drugs considered in this chapter are not likely to worsen hypertension.

IMPAIRED IMMUNITY

The prospect of certain drugs of abuse altering immunity is an important consideration for many abusers, not least those who are HIV positive or who have AIDS. A study in San Francisco, in which HIV-infected individuals were followed for six years, revealed that none of the drugs of abuse taken was associated with increased likelihood of progression to AIDS [46]. These drugs included: cannabis, opioids, alkyl nitrites, amphetamine derivatives, cocaine. This contrasts with a Scottish study suggesting that although other drugs of abuse had no effects, heroin could hasten progression to AIDS [47].

The potential for opioids to affect immunity has been studied in some detail. Endogenous opioids seem to have an immunoregulatory function in many species, including humans [48], and the administration of exogenous opioid may disrupt this process. The addition of morphine to cells infected with HIV and cultured *in vitro* results in increased replication of the virus [49]. A variety of signs of impaired immunity have been detected in both HIV-negative and HIV-positive patients taking methadone, including alterations in lymphocyte phenotype, suppressed lymphocyte function and reduced cytotoxic function of certain lymphocytes [50]. An analysis of the immunocompetence of 220 patients receiving daily methadone as maintenance treatment also revealed detrimental effects upon immunity regardless of HIV status. Specifically, the ratio of CD4 lymphocytes, which bolster immunity, to CD8 lymphocytes, which have a suppressor function, was reduced apparently due to increased CD8 numbers [51]. The study of 156 HIV-infected intravenous drug users in Scotland referred to above, found that those who continued to inject heroin were significantly more likely to progress to AIDS [47].

Alkyl nitrites are known to have detrimental effects upon lymphocytes *in vitro*. Both functional deficits and structural alterations have been observed which would be expected to reduce the effectiveness of lymphocytes if reproduced *in vivo* [52]. Some animal studies have shown no effect, others show a reduced helper T-lymphocyte level [53]. In humans, small studies have suggested that nitrite use can be associated with a decreased helper: suppressor T-lymphocyte ratio [54] or a decreased total lymphocyte count followed by an increase seven days later [55]. However, it is not clear whether these effects are clinically relevant in humans. Several studies have suggested that a history of nitrite abuse is one factor that can be associated with an increased risk of developing Kaposi's sarcoma in patients with AIDS [55–57]. In addition, nitrites might be converted to carcinogenic nitrosamines *in vivo* by mammalian metabolism. Although the case against alkyl nitrites cannot be said to be proven and it is largely circumstantial, it would be prudent for those who are immunosuppressed to avoid abusing them.

Cannabis has traditionally been held to possess immunosuppressive properties. However, the evidence for this is equivocal. *In vitro* studies using very high doses of cannabis have demonstrated adverse effects upon mammalian immunity but clinical studies have not demonstrated a convincing link [58].

It has been suggested that anabolic steroids might have immunosuppressant effects but the evidence for this is poor, being based on a very small number of case reports (see Chapter 10). Similarly it has been suggested anecdotally that ecstasy might have a mild immunosuppressant effect because many users claim to suffer from colds more frequently but there are no formal studies. One author suggests that this effect is due to the milieu in which ecstasy is taken: hot crowded dance floors, with lots of body contact, where colds and influenza are readily contracted [59]. Fatigue and loss of appetite induced by ecstasy could also increase susceptibility to these minor illnesses.

Regular smoking of any drug increases the risk of respiratory tract infections. In some cases contamination of the material with fungi has led to the development of fungal chest infections. Those who are immunosuppressed will be more prone to this effect of smoking and to infections derived from injection of non-sterile materials (see Chapter 2).

RENAL FAILURE

As with hepatic failure, one must consider the potential effects of the drug upon the disease and of the disease upon the elimination of the drug [60–62].

Nephrotoxicity

None of the drugs of abuse are commonly directly toxic to the kidney. However, certain drugs can cause acute myoglobinuric renal failure, secondary to rhabdomyolysis. This occurs when stimulants facilitate overexercise and then hyperpyrexia. The reaction is particularly associated with ecstasy but has also been reported with amphetamine and cocaine (see Chapter 6). There are two other pertinent ways in which drug abuse can be associated with rhabdomyolysis. Intra-arterial injection of some preparations can cause skeletal muscle ischaemia (see Chapter 2) and unconsciousness secondary to intoxication can lead to pressure-related muscle damage. If other organ systems are unaffected, the renal function will normalise within a few weeks.

Acute renal failure may occur subsequent to hypotension caused by overdoses of intravenous heroin. This usually resolves quickly.

Cocaine tends to have the opposite effect upon blood pressure. It can cause renal damage secondary to uncontrolled hypertension, usually in the form of nephrosclerosis or glomerulosclerosis.

Heroin-associated nephropathy has also been described but this now seems to be more rare than previously. It has been suggested that this is because the condition might have been due to heroin adulteration in the past and the drug is now much more pure at street level [62]. Alternatively, as many intravenous drug abusers have died early of AIDS or other infection, the condition may not have time to develop. Septicaemia itself can also cause acute renal failure. It can occur secondary to non-sterile injections.

Amyloidosis can arise as a result of chronic subcutaneous injection of drugs and this can in turn trigger a form of nephrotic syndrome. Antimuscarinic drugs can cause urinary retention.

Volatile substance abuse has rarely been associated with renal damage, not least because these compounds are excreted very rapidly. However, toluene is eliminated from the body more slowly and has been associated with renal tubular acidosis [63] and glomerulonephritis [64], although the latter has also been associated with other hydrocarbon solvents [31].

Drug accumulation in renal failure

With the exception of the opioids and ecstasy, none of the drugs of abuse considered in this chapter are eliminated renally to a great extent. It would therefore be anticipated that these drugs would not accumulate in patients with renal impairment. Ecstasy is mainly eliminated renally.

Morphine and heroin (which is converted to morphine), are metabolised to morphine-6-glucuronide which, although only produced in small quantities, is a very potent opioid agonist. It is known to accumulate in patients with renal failure, with potentially serious consequences, and so heroin should be used with extreme caution in renal failure. It would be important to stabilise any heroin-dependent individual with renal failure on a regular dose of methadone quickly rather than allow continued abuse of street heroin. Pethidine is metabolised to a neurotoxic derivative, norpethidine, which is eliminated renally. This metabolite accumulates in renal failure and causes excitation of the central nervous system (CNS) and even convulsions. The fentanyl-derived opioid designer drugs are probably eliminated hepatically, like the parent compound, and with inactive metabolites. These opioids should not, therefore, accumulate in renal impairment.

However, the situation is further complicated by the fact that patients with renal failure typically become more sensitive to the CNS effects of many drugs, probably because of the accumulation of urea. Consequently certain drugs of abuse may seem to exert more powerful effects. Although this field has not been studied adequately, increased sensitivity to CNS depressant drugs such as opioids, benzodiazepines and alcohol is widely recognised.

REFERENCES

1. Khalsa, M.E., Tashkin, D.P. and Perrochet, B. (1992) Smoked cocaine: patterns of use and pulmonary consequences. *J. Psychoact. Drugs*, **24**: 265–272.
2. Rubin, R.B. and Neugarten, J. (1990) Cocaine-associated asthma (letter). *Am. J. Med.* **88**: 438–439.
3. Suhl, J. and Gorelick, D.A. (1988) Pulmonary function in male free-base cocaine smokers (abstract). *Am. J. Resp. Dis.* **137**: 488.
4. Averbach, M., Casey, K.K. and Frank, E. (1996) Near-fatal status asthmaticus induced by nasal insufflation of cocaine. *South. Med. J.* **89**: 340–341.
5. Benson, M.K. and Bentley, A.M. (1995) Lung disease induced by drug addiction. *Thorax*, **50**: 1125–1127.
6. Rao, G. and Sloan, J.P. (1988) Alcohol-induced bronchospasm. *Arch. Emerg. Med.* **5**: 186–188.
7. Stockley, I.H. (1996) Theophylline + tobacco or cannabis smoking, in *Drug Interactions*, 4th Edn, The Pharmaceutical Press, London, pp. 802–803.
8. Anderson, K. (1986) Bronchospasm and intravenous street heroin (letter). *Lancet*, **i**: 1208.
9. Oliver, R.M. (1986) Bronchospasm and heroin inhalation (letter). *Lancet*, **i**: 915.
10. Stockley, I.H. (1996) Hypoglycaemic agents and alcohol, in *Drug Interactions*, 4th Edn, The Pharmaceutical Press, London, pp. 557–559.
11. Anon. (1994) Alcohol and hormones. *Alcohol Alert*, **26**: 1–2.
12. Campbell, R.K. (1986) Marijuana and diabetes. *Diabetes Educator*, **11**: 54.
13. Stockley, I.H. (1996) Hypoglycaemic agents + tobacco smoking, in *Drug Interactions*, 4th Edn, The Pharmaceutical Press, London, p. 591.
14. Stockley, I.H. (1996) Hypoglycaemic agents + anabolic steroids, in *Drug Interactions*, 4th Edn, The Pharmaceutical Press, London, pp. 559–560
15. Gold, M.A. and Gladstein, J. (1993) Substance use among adolescents with diabetes mellitus: preliminary findings. *J. Adolescent Health*, **14**: 80–84.

16. Alldredge, B.K., Lowenstein, D.H. and Simon, R.P. (1989) Seizures associated with recreational drug abuse. *Neurology*, **39**: 1037–1039.

17. Myers, J.A. and Earnest, M.P. (1984) Generalized seizures and cocaine abuse. *Neurology*, **34**: 675–676.

18. Choy-Kwong, M. and Lipton, R.B. (1989) Seizures in hospitalized cocaine users. *Neurology*, **39**: 425–427.

19. Jonsson, S., O'Meara, M. and Young, J.B. (1983) Acute cocaine poisoning: importance of treating seizures and acidosis. *Am. J. Med.* **75**: 1061–1064.

20. Ng, S.K.C., Brust, J.C.M., Hauser, W.A. and Susser, M. (1990) Illicit drug use and the risk of new-onset seizures. *Am. J. Epidemiol.* **132**: 47–57.

21. Gregory, R.E., Grossman, S. and Sheidler, V.R. (1992) Grand mal seizures associated with high-dose intravenous morphine infusions: incidence and possible etiology. *Pain*, **51**: 255–258.

22. Smith, N.T., Benthuysen, J.L., Bickford, R.G. *et al.* (1989) Seizures during opioid anesthetic induction – are they opioid-induced rigidity? *Anesthesiology*, **71**: 852–862.

23. Keeler, M.H. and Reifler, C.F. (1967) Grand mal convulsions subsequent to marijuana use. *Dis. Nerv. Syst.* **18**: 474–475.

24. Feeney, D.M. (1976) Marihuana use among epileptics (letter). *J. Am. Med. Assoc.* **235**: 1105.

25. Sofia, R.D., Soloman, T.A. and Barry, H. (1971) The anticonvulsant activity of delta-one tetrahydrocannabinol in mice. *Fed. Proc.* **13**: 305.

26. Consroe, P.F., Wood, G.C. and Buchsbaum, H. (1975) Anticonvulsant nature of marihuana smoking. *J. Am. Med. Assoc.* **234**: 306–307.

27. Carlini, E.A. and Cunha, J.M. (1981) Hypnotic and antiepileptic effects of cannabinol. *J. Clin. Pharmacol.* **21(suppl.)**: 417S–427S.

28. Stockley, I.H. (1996) Phenytoin + benzodiazepines, in *Drug Interactions*, 4th Edn, The Pharmaceutical Press, London, p. 341.

29. Farrell, G.C. (1994) *Drug-induced Liver Disease*, Churchill Livingstone, Edinburgh, pp. 288–289.

30. Baerg, R.D. and Kimberg, D.V. (1970) Centrilobular hepatic necrosis and acute renal failure in 'solvent sniffers'. *Ann. Intern. Med.* **73**: 713–720.

31. Marjot, R. and McLeod, A.A. (1989) Chronic non-neurological toxicity from volatile substance abuse. *Hum. Toxicol.* **8**: 301–306.

32. Ungvary, G., Tattai, E., Szeberenyi, S., Rodics, K., Lorincz, M. and Barcza, G. (1982) Effect of toluene exposure on the liver under different experimental conditions. *Exp. Mol. Pathol.* **36**: 347–360.

33. Farrell, G.C. (1994) *Drug-induced Liver Disease*, Churchill Livingstone, Edinburgh, pp. 236–239.

34. Kothur, R., Marsh Jr, F. and Posner, G. (1991) Liver function tests in nonparenteral cocaine users. *Arch. Intern. Med.* **151**: 1126–1128.

35. Wanless, I.R., Dore, S., Gopinath, N., Tan, J., Cameron, R. and Heathcote, E.J. (1990) Histopathology of cocaine hepatotoxicity: report of four patients. *Gastroenterology*, **98**: 497–501.

36. Perino, L.E., Warren, G.H. and Levine, J.S. (1987) Cocaine-induced hepatotoxicity in humans. *Gastroenterology*, **93**: 176–180.

37. Jover, R., Ponsoda, X., Gomez-Lechon, M.J., Herrero, C., Del Pino, J. and Castell, J.V. (1991) Potentiation of cocaine hepatotoxicity by ethanol in human hepatocytes. *Toxicol. Appl. Pharmacol.* **107**: 526–534.

38. Worner, T.M. (1994) Hepatotoxicity is not increased in alcoholics with positive urinary cocaine metabolites. *Drug Alcohol Dependence*, **35**: 191–195.

39. Trigueiro de Araujo, M.S., Gerard, F., Chossegros, P., Porto, L.C., Barlet, P. and Grimaud, J-A. (1990) Vascular hepatotoxicity related to heroin addiction. *Pathol. Anat. Histopathol.* **417**: 497–503.

40. Jover, R., Ponsoda, X., Gomez-Lechon, M.J. and Castell, J.V. (1992) Potentiation of heroin and methadone hepatotoxicity by ethanol: an in vitro study using cultured human hepatocytes. *Xenobiotica*, **22**: 471–478.

41. Brunt, P.W. and McGee, J.O'D. (1995) Chronic alcohol abuse: alimentary tract, pancreas and liver. *Medicine*, **23**: 54–60.

42. Farrell, G.C. (1994) *Drug-induced Liver Disease*, Churchill Livingstone, Edinburgh, pp. 177, 334–335.

43. Henry, J.A., Jeffreys, K.J. and Dawling, S. (1992) Toxicity and deaths from 3,4-methylenedioxymethamphetamine ('ecstasy'). *Lancet*, **340**: 384–387.

44. Shearman, J.D., Chapman, R.W.G., Satsangi, J., Ryley, N.G. and Weatherhead, S. (1992) Misuse of ecstasy (letter). *Br. Med. J.* **305**: 309.

45. Gorard, D.A., Davies, S.E. and Clark, M.L. (1992) Misuse of ecstasy (letter). *Br. Med. J.* **305**: 309.

46. DiFranco, M.J., Sheppard, H.W., Hunter, D.J., Tosteson, T.D. and Ascher, M.S. (1996) The lack of association of marijuana and other recreational drugs with progression to AIDS in the San Francisco men's health study. *Ann. Epidemiol.* **6**: 283–289.

47. Ronald, P.J.M., Robertson, J.R. and Elton, R.A. (1994) Continued drug use and other cofactors for progression to AIDS among injecting drug users. *AIDS*, **8**: 339–343.

48. Stefano, G.B., Scharrer, B., Smith, E.M. *et al.* (1996) Opioid and opiate immunoregulatory processes. *Crit. Rev. Immunol.* **16**: 109–144.

49. Scweitzer, C., Keller, F., Schmitt, F. *et al.* (1991) Morphine stimulates HIV replication in primary cultures of human Kuppffer cells. *Res. Virol.* **142**: 189–195.

50. Klimas, N.G., Blaney, N.T., Morgan, R.O. *et al.* (1991) Immune function and anti-HTLV-I/II status in anti-HIV-I-negative intravenous drug users receiving methadone. *Am. J. Med.* **90**: 163–170.

51. Carballo-Dieguez, A., Sahs, J., Goetz, R., El Sadr, W., Sorell, S. and Gorman, J. (1994) The effect of methadone on immunological parameters among HIV-positive and HIV-negative drug users. *Am. J. Drug Alcohol Abuse*, **20**: 317–329.
52. Jacobs, R.F., Marmer, D.J., Steele, R.W. and Hogue, T.R. (1983) Cellular immunotoxicity of amyl nitrite. *J. Toxicol.* **20**: 421–449.
53. Haverkos, H.W. and Dougherty, J. (1988) Health hazards of nitrite inhalants. *Am. J. Med.* **84**: 479–482.
54. Goedert, J.J., Neuland, C.Y., Wallen, W.C. *et al.* (1982) Amyl nitrite may alter T-lymphocytes in homosexual men. *Lancet*, **i**: 412–416.
55. Lange, W.R. and Fralich, J. (1989) Nitrite inhalants: promising and discouraging news (editorial). *Br. J. Addict.* **84**: 121–123.
56. Marmor, M., Friedman-Kien, A.E., Laubenstein, L. *et al.* (1982) Risk factors for Kaposi's sarcoma in homosexual men. *Lancet*, **i**: 1083–1087.
57. Mathur-Wagh, U., Mildvan, D. and Senie, R.T., (1985) Follow-up at four and a half years on homosexual men with generalized lymphadenopathy (letter). *N. Engl. J. Med.* **313**: 1541–1543.
58. Hollister, L.E. (1992) Marijuana and immunity. *J. Psychoactive Drugs*, **24**: 159–164.
59. Saunders, N. (1995) *Ecstasy and the Dance Culture*, BPC Wheatons, England, p. 78.
60. Levitan, D. (1982) Effects of drug abuse on the kidney. *Dialysis Transpl.* **11**: 885–886.
61. Ghodse, A.H. (1993) Substance abuse leading to renal damage. *Prescribers' J.* **33**: 151–155.
62. Bakir, A.A. and Dunes, G. (1996) Drugs of abuse and renal disease. *Curr. Opin. Nephrol. Hypertension*, **5**: 122–126.
63. Voigts, A. and Kaufman, C.E. (1983) Acidosis and other metabolic abnormalities associated with paint sniffing. *South. Med. J.* **76**: 443–447.
64. Venkataraman, G. (1981) Renal damage and glue sniffing (letter). *Br. Med. J.* **283**: 1467.

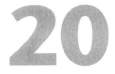

Drugs in pregnancy and breast-feeding

It is as natural to die as to be born; and to a little infant, perhaps, the one is as painful as the other.
Sir Francis Bacon, 1561–1626, *Essays*, 'Of Death'.

DRUG ABUSE IN PREGNANCY

It is particularly difficult to study drug abuse in human pregnancy. There are a number of reasons for this.

- Recruitment. Suitable women may be difficult to identify because they may feel guilty about their drug taking, be afraid to tell health-care staff about illegal drug use and be frightened of reproaches from relatives should this come to light.
- Confounding. The lifestyle of many women who abuse drugs may already predispose them to an adverse pregnancy outcome, e.g. living conditions, general health, reproductive health, nutritional status and socioeconomic group. Separating environmental and personal confounders is particularly difficult when trying to follow-up drug-exposed infants after birth.
- Multi-drug use. It is almost impossible to study any single drug of abuse in complete isolation because multi-drug use is common. Tobacco and alcohol alone are frequently consumed by those who abuse street drugs, and these are known to have adverse effects upon the foetus.
- Identification. Many drug abusers do not know exactly what they are taking, either in terms of identity (due to adulteration) or in terms of dose (due to impurity and dilution).

- Collecting data. Usually studies rely on maternal recall of the extent and nature of drug use during pregnancy and this may not be reliable.
- Changing use. The pattern of use may change during the pregnancy. Mothers may increase or decrease dose or frequency.

Apart from the pharmacological effects that are directly specific to the developing foetus, drugs of abuse can affect the foetus in other ways. Those who inject drugs during pregnancy are at increased risk of becoming infected with HIV if they share injecting equipment. This can be passed on to the foetus. Any serious drug-related maternal illness may threaten the health of mother or foetus during pregnancy, e.g. seizures due to cocaine, hyperpyrexia due to ecstasy, liver damage due to alcohol, septicaemia due to non-sterile injection and accidents due to intoxication with any drug.

Perhaps the most difficult area of all to study is the effect of *in utero* drug exposure upon later childhood development. Subtle drug-induced neurological damage to the developing foetus, which may not be noticeable at birth, could result in physical, emotional, psychiatric or behavioural problems which might only be apparent later in life when the association with maternal drug abuse can no longer be made. Once out of the womb, there are a large number of potentially confounding variables which can interfere with study in this area.

Clearly it is preferable if women who abuse drugs can stop taking them before conception. However, in reality this does not occur because pregnancies are unplanned, women do not understand the risks of continued abuse or because mothers are physically dependent and cannot stop without support. In these situations it can be helpful to inform mothers of the potential risks to their babies. This chapter aims to provide this information in a reasonably succinct way.

DRUG ABUSE IN BREAST-FEEDING WOMEN

All drugs pass into human milk to some extent and, ideally of course, drugs of abuse should not be taken whilst breast-feeding. Unfortunately, for most drugs of abuse there is very little information available on the extent of drug passage into milk and the effects upon the infant. Most of the data comes from case histories in the medical literature and, as with most biological and pharmacological processes, there is a potentially large inter-patient variation in the kinetics of drugs in lactating women. The small number of reports may therefore be unrepresentative. Three basic factors which affect the extent of penetration into human milk are the following.

1. Drugs that are highly protein bound in plasma tend to cross into milk in much smaller amounts than those which are not bound so extensively.
2. Fat-soluble drugs can concentrate into the lipid phase of milk (although this phase is a small proportion of the total volume).
3. Weak bases tend to concentrate in milk because it is slightly acidic relative to plasma.

Most of the drugs of abuse considered here are largely metabolised in the liver. Liver metabolism can be markedly deficient in babies, especially if they are premature. This may allow accumulation. Babies are also more sensitive than adults to most drugs that act on the central nervous system (CNS) and, again, prematures are especially sensitive to this effect. However, when deciding whether it is wise for a nursing mother taking drugs to breast feed, it is important to consider other factors besides milk penetration by the drug. One could take the view of the American Academy of Pediatrics that nursing mothers should not ingest any drugs of abuse whilst breast feeding because drugs could be hazardous to the infant and to the physical and emotional health of the mother [1]. This is obviously the ideal situation but it is unrealistic because in practice some women are dependent upon drugs or will simply want to take them regardless, and will have to decide whether to breast feed or not. It is vital that each case is assessed individually. Breast feeding has a variety of important benefits to the baby, including increased mother–infant bonding, increased immunity to infection (and perhaps other diseases) and balanced nutritional intake. A decision not to breast feed should be made with due consideration for these factors and should also take into account that the alternative to breast-feeding (bottle feeding) is a more time-consuming option which requires attention to sterility and careful preparation. In addition bottle feeding can be costly. Some mothers may not be able to cope with bottle feeding for a variety of reasons and in certain circumstances it may be preferable to encourage breast-feeding despite the baby being exposed to a street drug in the mother's milk, i.e. it may be the 'least worst option'.

Certain measures can be taken to limit the baby's exposure to drugs if a nursing mother does take drugs of abuse and breast feed. It is obviously helpful if the mother can reduce the dose of drug taken. The mother should also try and take the drug immediately after feeding and avoid feeding while intoxicated, so that the baby is not exposed to the highest maternal level of drug. If possible the drug should be taken at night after the last feed and nursing avoided thereafter until the next morning. In some situations the mother may be able to express and save breast milk during a time of the day when drug exposure is low and administer this later when infant exposure to drug would be higher if milk was given directly from the breast.

In most cases there are no data on the long-term effects upon the infant of exposure to drugs of abuse in human milk. Since drugs of abuse all act upon the CNS to some extent, it is possible that there could be adverse effects upon mental development, behaviour or psychiatric health but this is a very under-researched area. It might be anticipated that regular taking of drugs of abuse might impair parenting skills but this has also not be studied.

The details below are a summary of the clinical data that have been published.

ALCOHOL

Pregnancy

Continued heavy drinking is most likely to affect the foetus, and the worst effects are seen in alcoholics but the effects of alcohol in pregnancy are probably dose-dependent. In terms of damage to the foetus, it is particularly difficult to separate the contribution made directly by high levels of ethanol from other aspects of the alcoholic's lifestyle. For example, alcoholics often have a very poor diet and are more likely to smoke. Despite this it is generally believed that alcohol is teratogenic. Foetal alcohol syndrome (FAS) has been identified in babies born to alcoholics and those who regularly drink heavily, although many of these women are delivered of apparently healthy babies. FAS has the following characteristics:

- intra-uterine growth retardation (including reduced weight at birth and decreased head circumference);
- characteristic facial changes;
- neurological defects (especially reduced mental ability and brain anomalies);
- congenital abnormalities (especially heart damage, limb malformations, genitourinary defects).

In addition, FAS is associated with delayed mental development, retardation, low IQ and various behavioural problems later in life. Reduced growth rate and small size can also continue into childhood, although facial changes may diminish with time. The FAS has been associated with 'heavy drinking' but the precise definition of this in terms of the quantity of alcohol required is unclear. FAS probably represents the worst end of a spectrum of dose-related damage that alcohol can cause to the foetus. Babies born to women who drink smaller amounts of ethanol than a chronic alcoholic can still show evidence of harm such as minor anomalies, growth deficiency and behavioural problems.

Moderate to heavy alcohol use in pregnancy is also associated with an increased risk of prematurity, miscarriage, stillbirth and spontaneous abortion. Some neonates appear to be delivered with CNS depression due to alcohol and experience withdrawal reactions. Symptoms include tremors, irritability, apnoea, restlessness, hypertonia and agitation. These usually appear within a few hours of birth and resolve within a few days. There is a greater risk of perinatal mortality amongst babies born to alcoholics.

There is no particular evidence that a single occasional drink is associated with an adverse effect upon pregnancy outcome but a 'safe' level of drinking in pregnancy has not been established. It is also not clear whether alcohol can cause damage at any stage of pregnancy or whether there are periods of lesser risk. As a result it would be best to avoid all alcohol during pregnancy until studies are available which can accurately estimate the risk to the foetus of low intake.

Breast-feeding

Alcohol passes into breast milk, although acetaldehyde, the major pharmacologically active metabolite, does not. Very large maternal doses caused a reversible 'Cushing's syndrome' like effect in one breast-fed infant [2] and 'drunkenness' in another baby [3]. However, these are isolated reports. A more ubiquitous property of alcohol is its ability to inhibit milk ejection in a dose-dependent way by blocking the release of oxytocin from the pituitary in response to suckling [4]. A high intake of alcohol can inhibit milk flow completely. When breast feeding occurs immediately after consuming an alcoholic drink, the infant is found to consume only about three-quarters of the amount of milk which it would do otherwise [4]. The precise reasons for this are unclear but it may be that alcohol imparts a disagreeable taste to the milk.

One study has shown that regular alcohol intake can adversely affect motor development at one year [5]. One drink a day had only slight effects, occasional drinking had no effect. The impairment was more marked if more than six drinks a day were taken during nursing. No adverse mental effects were reported.

Notwithstanding these effects, it is generally considered acceptable to consume small amounts of alcohol while breast-feeding. However, it is easy to avoid breast feeding for one or two hours after a single alcoholic drink – thus reducing infant exposure – and this should be recommended.

AMPHETAMINES

Pregnancy

Amphetamine is not thought to cause congenital abnormalities. Studies of cohorts of women taking the drug do not reveal an increased risk. When the participants in such studies are summated, the published cohort studies to date include about 3000 women. However, one case-control study (where a link is sought retrospectively between babies with a given anomaly) suggested that amphetamine could be a contributory factor to the development of congenital heart disease [6]. But case-control studies are subject to a variety of confounders and are less reliable than cohort studies. A larger case-control study (219 patients) and a prospective study of 50 patients failed to establish a link with congenital heart disease [7].

Amphetamine is known to cause maternal anorexia (which can result in relative malnutrition), hypertension and reduced blood flow to the placenta. Intrauterine growth retardation and foetal hypoxia are possible adverse effects upon the neonate as a result of these actions. Amphetamine abuse is probably associated with low birth weight, prematurity and increased perinatal mortality. However, these effects have been inadequately studied. Some studies suggest that maternal amphetamine abuse near term is associated with neonatal drowsiness and even withdrawal symptoms but information on this is scant. The limited studies of childhood development suggest little difference between amphetamine exposed infants and the general population at one year of age.

There is no information at all on the actions of ecstasy in human pregnancy. At the present time one can only assume that the effects would be similar to those of amphetamine.

Breast-feeding

There is only one detailed case report in the literature of amphetamine administration to a breast-feeding mother. Milk from a woman receiving 20 mg of dexamphetamine daily for therapeutic reasons was analysed [8].

The drug was found to be much more concentrated in milk than in plasma. Despite this, no adverse effects were reported in the baby who was periodically assessed for 2 years. Similarly, a review of 103 infants receiving milk from mothers who took amphetamines (various forms and doses) revealed no acute side effects in the recipients [9]. Theoretically, amphetamines might be anticipated to cause stimulation (irritability, poor sleep pattern) or sedation (poor feeding) in infants. On the whole, children tend to be sedated by amphetamines rather than stimulated.

Although the effects upon lactation have not been studied specifically, high doses of amphetamine do suppress prolactin secretion in patients with hyperprolactinaemia [10]. If this effect were to occur in lactating women the drug might reduce milk production. There is no information at all on any of the amphetamine derivatives such as ecstasy and methamphetamine in lactation.

ANABOLIC STEROIDS

Pregnancy

There is no information on anabolic steroid abuse in pregnancy. When the therapeutic drugs testosterone or danazol are used inadvertently in human pregnancy each can be associated with virilisation of the genitalia of female foetuses. These drugs are related to anabolic steroids but therapeutically are used in much smaller amounts than the anabolic steroids used by abusers. No adverse effects have been described in male foetuses.

Breast-feeding

Anabolic steroid use in breast-feeding does not appear to have been studied. However, the androgenic properties of this group of steroids are known to reduce breast size when taken chronically and in this situation impaired milk production would seem likely. Anabolic steroids are lipid-soluble so milk penetration should be anticipated. These drugs might cause virilisation of girls exposed to them via breast milk.

BENZODIAZEPINES

Pregnancy

Most studies suggest that benzodiazepines (BZDs) are not likely to cause congenital malformations. Other studies suggesting a teratogenic effect have not demonstrated a consistent pattern of abnormalities. Very limited data suggest a link to dysmorphism but if this is an effect of BZDs it must be rare (a specific link to cleft palate has also been suggested but not been proven).

During prolonged maternal administration, BZDs may accumulate in the foetus at a greater concentration than in the mother. After birth the drug may remain in the newborn for a long time due to the immaturity of the neonatal liver resulting in sedation, lethargy, reduced muscle tone, hypothermia and poor feeding. These effects can be most noticeable when a dose of BZD is given close to birth and have been referred to as the 'floppy infant syndrome'. Withdrawal reactions can occur if BZD exposure *in utero* was chronic and are very similar to those described for neonatal opioid withdrawal (see Table 20.1 and below).

Chronic BZD use during pregnancy has been associated with low birth weight in one small study.

Breast-feeding

Although all the BZDs are excreted into breast milk to some degree, small doses for a short period are probably acceptable in breast-feeding mothers. However, the very large doses used by those who abuse them at street level could have a detrimental effect on the baby who is breast fed, by causing sedation. The BZDs are cleared hepatically and so would be expected to accumulate in babies due to their immature metabolism. Consequently, the worst effects of sedation might not be seen for several days after starting regular administration of maternal BZDs. The effects of this sedation are unknown so it would be better for regular high-dose BZD abusers to avoid breast-feeding. Those taking BZDs for therapeutic reasons should be encouraged to take a short course only, and the baby monitored for sedation.

CAFFEINE

Pregnancy

Studies involving several thousand women have shown that caffeine is unlikely to cause congenital anomalies at normal intake. There is less information on very high caffeine consumption. Human studies suggest that high doses might be associated with spontaneous abortion or reduced birth weight but this has not been proven. Work involving monkeys has reported an increased incidence of miscarriages and still-births at high dose. Reversible cardiac arrhythmias have been described in the human foetus and newborn after exposure to very high caffeine doses [11]. In 1988, eight newborns with apparent caffeine withdrawal symptoms were described. Their mothers had consumed large amounts of caffeine. Symptoms included jitteriness and vomiting [12].

Breast-feeding

Caffeine is commonly taken by breast-feeding women and there are no apparent adverse effects upon the nursing infant at normal levels of intake. Caffeine is used therapeutically at a dose of up to 10 mg/kg/day (of base) to treat neonatal apnoea. This is a considerably higher dose than could be achieved by drinking caffeinated beverages and it is not associated with significant side effects.

CANNABIS

Pregnancy

Cannabis is commonly abused in pregnancy. Some studies have shown that it increases the likelihood of premature delivery especially in heavy users but not all studies have confirmed this. Most suggest that this is not likely to be a significant effect when demographic factors are taken into account. It has been suggested that cannabis can decrease *in utero* growth leading to small birth weight babies. However, again, the majority of studies do not support this.

There are case reports and small studies in the medical literature suggesting that cannabis might have a teratogenic effect but the diverse array of adverse foetal effects mitigates against a drug-related effect. In addition, in many of these studies potentially confounding variables were not excluded. If cannabis does cause foetal malformations then the effect must be rare and occur only at high doses because most studies do not reveal a teratogenic effect.

A study in 1989 suggested that foetal exposure to cannabis was associated with an increased risk for developing childhood leukaemia [13]. Ten out of 204 exposed cases had leukaemia, compared to only one of 203 controls. The leukaemia developed at a younger age than normal in the cannabis group (at about 38 months). This study requires confirmation.

The effects of *in utero* cannabis exposure upon infant behaviour has not been studied adequately. So far results suggest that newborns that were exposed to cannabis in the womb may show increased startle responses, tremor and visual response abnormalities but the significance of these are unknown. Follow-up of these babies at one year showed no differences compared to controls. Other studies in older children have given equivocal results.

Breast-feeding

Delta-9-tetrahydrocannabinol (THC) passes into breast milk when smoked or when given orally for therapeutic reasons (dronabinol) and may even be concentrated in it. Despite this, two detailed case reports provided no evidence of acute adverse reactions in the infant [14]. However, given the nature of cannabis and its actions in humans, which are more subtle than many of the other illicit substances, any effects in babies would probably be difficult to identify. As with tobacco (see below), the baby may be exposed to the drug via passive inhalation of smoke as well as via milk, so parents should avoid smoking in the same room as babies. The long-term effects upon infants have not been studied adequately. One study of 27 babies exposed to cannabis via breast milk revealed no mental or physical differences between exposed babies and controls at one year of age [15]. By contrast, another study showed a deficient motor development at one year in cannabis-exposed infants [16].

In animals cannabis may reduce lactation by suppressing prolactin secretion [17]. A similar effect upon prolactin has been observed in non-breast feeding women [18] but this has not been studied in lactating women.

COCAINE

Pregnancy

Cocaine has potent vasoconstricting and hypertensive properties and these may be important in the aetiology of many of the adverse effects noted in pregnancy. Cocaine can restrict blood flow to the uterus, cause foetal hypoxia and trigger uterine contractions. Foetal CNS infarction and other brain anomalies have also been reported and may be related to cocaine-induced brain haemorrhage or ischaemia. Persistent neonatal arterial hypertension is also known.

Cocaine has been associated with an increased incidence of spontaneous abortion, stillbirth, prematurity and abruptio placentae, which is often linked to foetal death.

Decreased neonatal weight and size, including decreased head circumference, are associated with *in utero* exposure to cocaine, perhaps due to reduced oxygen supply to the foetus. Limited evidence suggests that these babies can make good this decreased weight and size in early infancy.

It has been claimed that cocaine can cause a wide variety of congenital defects but these effects have either been reported from small studies or are described as defects for which there is only a small increased risk in larger studies. It is very difficult to ascertain which of these are true drug-related effects. Gut, genitourinary, skull and heart defects are most commonly described and many are attributed to cocaine's effects upon foetal circulation. On the whole cocaine probably has some teratogenic effects but it is not a highly teratogenic substance.

Babies may be irritable at birth and exhibit symptoms such as: tremor, hypertension, abnormal reflexes, tachypnoea, autonomic instability, vomiting, diarrhoea, seizures and poor feeding. Foetuses exposed to cocaine are at increased risk of perinatal death and some studies also reveal an association with sudden infant death syndrome (SIDS) but not all studies have confirmed this link.

Cocaine may be associated with developmental delay and mental retardation in infants born to cocaine-abusing women but this has not been studied adequately enough at present to allow definite conclusions to be made.

Breast-feeding

Cocaine intoxication has been reported in one infant receiving milk from a woman who had taken cocaine [19]. The baby experienced tachycardia, tachypnoea, hypertension, irritability and tremor. The infant's urine contained cocaine and metabolites. Young babies are relatively deficient in the plasma esterase enzymes needed to metabolise cocaine.

Although only one case report is available, the fact that it describes an adverse effect suggests that cocaine should not be used during breast-feeding.

LSD

Pregnancy

Of the commonly abused illicit substances, LSD has been studied the least in human pregnancy. There are several case reports in the medical literature which ascribe various congenital anomalies to LSD administration but there is no consistent pattern to these, rendering an association unlikely. All of the human studies are small. The evidence from these does not support a link between maternal LSD use and foetal malformations or other adverse pregnancy outcome but these data are limited. Research into the long-term effects of *in utero* exposure to LSD has not been conducted.

Breast-feeding

The use of LSD during lactation has never been reported in the medical literature. Consequently, use in breast-feeding should be avoided because the effects upon the infant are completely unknown. LSD is a very potent psychoactive compound even in small doses.

OPIOIDS

Pregnancy

Opioids are perhaps second only to cocaine as the most extensively studied drugs of abuse in human pregnancy. Although not all authorities are in agreement over the precise effects of taking opioids in pregnancy, the information presented here is that which most agree upon.

The daily administration of heroin or methadone during pregnancy is associated with increased rates of prematurity, low birth weight and small neonatal size. Reduced head circumference has particularly been noted. There is also an increased perinatal mortality. Several studies have suggested that there is an increased risk of SIDS amongst babies exposed to opioids *in utero*. The incidence could be as high as 4 per cent. Opioids are not thought to cause congenital abnormalities.

Preschool children who were exposed to opioids in the womb may exhibit a range of problems which have been attributed to drug exposure. The smaller head size noted at birth in some individuals may be persistent. Children may also show reduced growth and increased abnormal behaviour compared to their peers. Behavioural problems observed include hyperactivity, increased aggression and decreased inhibitions.

It has been argued that all of the effects discussed so far, except reduced newborn weight and size, are due more to the mother's or parents' lifestyle (living conditions, general health, diet, personality) than to the direct effects of opioids. Although this may be true, in practice it is extraordinarily difficult to separate environmental effects from pharmacological ones. One recent small study has suggested that moving opioid-exposed children away from their dependent parents at an early age, to foster or adoptive parents, may eliminate preschool behavioural differences [20].

Withdrawal reactions are common in neonates exposed to opioids throughout the third trimester. The majority are affected to some degree. Some authors feel that symptoms are worse in babies born to women receiving methadone than in those taking heroin. The typical symptoms are similar to those experienced in adults undergoing withdrawal (see Table 20.1).

Table 20.1 Withdrawal symptoms after *in utero* exposure to opioids

- Hypertonia, hyperreflexia, tremor
- Hyperactivity, irritability, poor sleeping pattern, decreased sleep
- Diarrhoea
- Tachypnoea, rhinorrhoea, yawning, hiccups, sneezing, apnoea
- Poor feeding, weight loss or failure to gain weight
- Fever
- High-pitched cry
- Lacrimation

Seizures can occur but these are often a later complication. They are probably more common in methadone exposed babies and occur typically at about 10 days after birth.

Withdrawal symptoms may be present at birth but, if not, onset usually occurs within 24 to 48 hours for babies born of heroin-dependent mothers and within two to seven days for babies exposed to methadone. Sometimes the peak intensity of symptoms can be delayed by as much as 10 to 14 days. The acute symptoms may persist for several weeks but usually these abate within three weeks for those exposed to heroin; the time course of methadone's effects is much more variable. Subacute symptoms such as sleeping problems, irritability and poor feeding may last for up to six months in some cases. It is generally believed, although not conclusively proven, that the intensity of neonatal withdrawal symptoms is related to maternal opioid dose. If possible, therefore, opioid intake should be gradually reduced during pregnancy. Babies born to mothers taking 20 mg of methadone per day or less seem to fare better than those exposed to greater doses.

Breast-feeding

The effects of heroin abuse in breast-feeding have not been investigated in recent times. Morphine does pass into breast milk in small amounts and the results of single dose studies suggest that when given for therapeutic effect, small doses are probably not a significant problem in breast feeding. The morphine in breast milk would be subject to the baby's first-pass liver metabolism which, although not studied in this age group, is quite extensive in adults. However, the effects on the breast-fed baby of maternal chronic administration of large doses of opioids is not known.

The American Academy of Pediatrics (AAP) states that tremors, restlessness, vomiting and poor feeding have occurred in infants receiving opioids in breast milk but these could be the result of withdrawal from *in utero* exposure [1]. Some have even advocated that mothers taking opioids should breast feed in order to prevent neonatal withdrawal from *in utero* exposure to opioids but this is a rather 'hit and miss' approach. Neonates are notoriously sensitive to opioids and metabolise them very slowly, so accumulation is possible. Methadone, which has a long half-life in adults, could be particularly liable to accumulate in babies but the concentration in milk seems to be less than that in maternal plasma. The AAP considers that methadone administration during nursing is not likely to be harmful to the infant if the mother takes no more than 20 mg per day. This is a rather unhelpful limit because very few patients take such a small maintenance dose.

In adults, certain opioids have a very limited bioavailability when given orally and so absorption of these from breast milk in the infant's gut may similarly be limited. Such drugs include buprenorphine and fentanyl. If it were possible to stabilise nursing mothers on maintenance doses of buprenorphine rather than methadone this may be preferable.

Opioids are given therapeutically to babies from time to time in very small doses and, apart from causing CNS depression and constipation, they do not appear to be intrinsically harmful. In overdose, excessive sedation and respiratory depression can occur. In practical terms, one would wish to monitor any baby for signs of sedation if a woman taking moderate to large doses of opioids wished to breast feed. Furthermore, one should be aware that when breast feeding stops the baby could experience withdrawal symptoms.

TOBACCO

Pregnancy

Tobacco smoking is associated with reduced oxygen supply and blood flow to the foetus. The following adverse effects are linked to smoking in pregnancy: spontaneous abortion, low birth weight, premature birth and increased perinatal mortality (including SIDS). All of these effects are more likely in women who are heavy smokers. The incidence is markedly reduced in women who cease smoking before the end of the first trimester. Although still rare, smoking increases the risk of congenital limb reduction defects [28]; other than this it has been difficult to associate smoking convincingly with teratogenic effects. However, tobacco smoking is associated with a twofold increase in risk of ectopic pregnancy.

Abnormal behaviour and impairment of intellectual development may persist into childhood but these effects are generally mild and the environmental contributions to them cannot be separated from the direct effect of tobacco smoking. The effects of reduced growth are usually overcome in early infancy.

Breast-feeding

The AAP states that shock, vomiting, diarrhoea, tachycardia, restlessness and insomnia have been reported in babies when tobacco was smoked by the mother during nursing [1], although this is probably based on one case report [3]. Nicotine can be concentrated in milk and has been reported to cause infantile colic [21,22]. The baby is exposed to nicotine partly via breast milk and partly via passive inhalation of smoke while the mother or others smoke near to the infant. Passive smoking is associated with increased respiratory tract infections. Nicotine can also lower prolactin levels so nursing mothers may find that they stop feeding sooner than non-smokers [22].

Mothers should not smoke just before feeding to reduce infant exposure to peak milk levels of nicotine; they should also avoid smoking near the baby and should try and reduce consumption if possible.

VOLATILE SUBSTANCE ABUSE

Pregnancy

Volatile substances can cause hypoxia so theoretically they could reduce oxygen supply to the foetal brain; however this has not been studied. Five cases of maternal renal tubular acidosis during pregnancy have been described in known heavy abusers of toluene; in three of the newborns delivered to these women there was growth retardation and in two of these hyperchloraemic acidosis [23].

Various studies of occupational exposure to solvents have been performed [24–26]. These have reported differing results depending upon the solvent involved and the extent of exposure. Taken as a whole they do not support a strong link between occupational exposure to solvents and adverse pregnancy outcome. Some studies claim an increased risk of congenital defects but there is no consistent pattern to the anomalies claimed and many studies show no association. Similarly, some studies have shown an increased risk of spontaneous abortion but others have not.

In 1996, a team of researchers in Canada suggested that volatile substance abuse can be associated with a neonatal withdrawal syndrome which may respond to treatment with phenobarbitone [27]. The syndrome was identified and treated in 32 babies born over a four-year period. The syndrome was characterised by a high pitched cry, lack of sleep, tremor, hypotonia, poor feeding and a hyperactive Moro reflex. Treatment was typically initiated about 24 hours after birth and lasted for approximately six days. The authors stated that the aroma of solvents in mother or baby may be a marker for this syndrome.

Breast-feeding

Volatile substance abuse in lactating women has not been studied but the very short half-lives of most volatile substances suggest that breast-feeding should not cause problems for the infant unless it occurs whilst the mother is actually intoxicated.

REFERENCES

1. Committee on Drugs (1994) The transfer of drugs and other chemicals into human milk. *Pediatrics*, **93**: 137–150.
2. Binkiewicz, A., Robinson, M.J. and Senior, B. (1978) Pseudo-Cushing syndrome caused by alcohol in breast milk. *J. Pediatr.* **93**: 965–967.
3. Bisdom, W. (1937) Alcohol and nicotine poisoning in nurslings. *J. Am. Med. Assoc.* **109**: 178.
4. Cobo, E. (1973) Effect of different doses of ethanol on the milk ejecting reflex in lactating women. *Am. J. Obstet. Gynecol.* **115**: 817–821.
5. Little, R.E., Anderson, K.W., Ervin, C.H., Worthington-Roberts, B. and Clarren, S.K. (1989) Maternal alcohol use during breast feeding and infant mental and motor development at one year. *N. Engl. J. Med.* **321**: 425–430.
6. Nora, J.J., Vargo, T.A., Nora, A.H., Love, K.E. and McNamara, D.G. (1970) Dexamphetamine: a possible environmental trigger in cardiovascular malformations. *Lancet*, **i**: 1290–1291.
7. Nora, J.J., McNamara, D.G. and Fraser, F.C. (1967) Dexamphetamine sulphate and human malformations. *Lancet*, **i**: 570–571.
8. Steiner, E., Villen, T., Hallberg, M. and Rane, A. (1984) Amphetamine secretion in breast milk. *Eur. J. Clin. Pharmacol.* **27**: 123–124.
9. Ayd (Jr), F.J. (1973) Excretion of psychotropic drugs in human breast milk. *Int. Drug Ther. News Bull.* **8**: 33–40.
10. DeLeo, V., Cella, S.G. and Camanni, F. (1983) Prolactin lowering effect of amphetamine in normoprolactinemic subjects and in physiological and pathological hyperprolactinaemia. *Horm. Metab. Res.* **15**: 439–443.
11. Oei, S.G., Vosters, R.P.L. and van der Hagen, N.L.J. (1989) Fetal arrhythmia caused by excessive intake of caffeine by pregnant women. *Br. Med. J.* **298**: 568.

12. McGowan, J.D., Altman, R.E. and Kanto, W.P. (1988) Neonatal withdrawal symptoms after chronic maternal ingestion of caffeine. *South. Med. J.* **81**: 1092.

13. Robison, L.L., Buckley, J.D., Daigle, A.E., Wells, R., Benjamin, D., Arthur, D.C. and Hammond, G.D. (1989) Maternal drug use and risk of childhood nonlymphoblastic leukaemia among offspring: an epidemiologic investigation implicating marijuana. *Cancer*, **63**: 1904–1911.

14. Perez-Reges, M. and Wall, M.E. (1982) Presence of tetrahydrocannabinol in human milk. *N. Engl. J. Med.* **307**: 819–820.

15. Tennes, K., Avitable, N., Blackard, C., Boyles, C., Hassoun, B., Holmes, L. and Kreye, M. (1985) Marijuana: prenatal and postnatal exposure in the human. *NIDA Res. Monogr.* **59**: 48–60.

16. Astley, S.J. and Little, R.E. (1990) Maternal marijuana use during lactation and infant development at one year. *Neurotoxicol. Teratol.* **12**: 161–168.

17. Haclerode, J. (1980) The effect of marijuana on reproduction and development. *NIDA Res. Monogr.* **31**: 137–166.

18. Mendelson, J.H., Mello, N.K. and Elingboe, J. (1985) Acute effects of marijuana smoking on prolactin levels in human females. *J. Pharmacol. Exp. Ther.* **123**: 220–222.

19. Chasnoff, I.J., Lewis, D.E. and Squires, L. (1987) Cocaine intoxication in a breast-fed infant. *Pediatrics*, **80**: 836–838.

20. Fishmann, R.H.B. (1996) Normal development after prenatal heroin. *Lancet*, **347**: 1397.

21. Said, G., Patois, E. and Lellouch, J. (1984) Infantile colic and parental smoking. *Br. Med. J.* **289**: 660.

22. Matheson, I. and Rivrud, G.N. (1989) The effect of smoking on lactation and infantile colic. *J. Am. Med. Assoc.* **261**: 42–43.

23. Goodwin, T.M. (1988) Toluene abuse and renal tubular acidosis in pregnancy. *J. Obstet. Gynecol.* **71**: 715–718.

24. Bentur, Y. and Koren, G. (1991) The three most common exposures reported by pregnant women: an update. *Am. J. Obstet. Gynecol.* **165**: 429–437.

25. Windham, G.C., Shusterman, D., Swan, S.H., Fenster, L. and Eskenazi, B. (1991) Exposure to organic solvents and adverse pregnancy outcome. *Am. J. Indust. Med.* **20**: 241–259.

26. Ahlborg, G. (1990) Pregnancy outcome among women working in laundries and dry-cleaning shops using tetrachloroethylene. *Am. J. Indust. Med.* **17**: 567–575.

27. Tenenbein, M., Casiro, O.G., Seshia, M.M.K. and Debooy, V.D. (1996) Neonatal withdrawal from maternal volatile substance abuse. *Arch. Dis. Child.* **74**: F204–F207.

28. Källén, K. (1997) Maternal smoking during pregnancy and limb reduction malformations in Sweden. *Am. J. Pub. Health* **87**: 29–32.

Appendix A

Pharmacists involved in schemes to supply clean syringes and needles

The Council of the Royal Pharmaceutical Society has issued the following guidelines for pharmacists who elect to become involved in schemes to exchange clean syringes and needles for contaminated equipment used by injecting substance and drug misusers.

1. Normally schemes will be promoted by health authorities and local pharmaceutical committees. In other cases the existing facilities should be researched and the pharmacist should consult the local pharmaceutical committee (area pharmaceutical committee), the local medical committee (area medical committee) and any local drug abuse teams and clinics in order to establish the need for pharmacists to take part.
2. The supply of syringes and needles and the receipt of used equipment should be dealt with by the pharmacist and supplies should always be accompanied by advice and encouragement to make use of any local drug advisory services. Approved leaflets from health education agencies, local drug dependency clinics or 'walk-in centres' should be available.
3. All clients requesting syringes and needles should be encouraged to return any used equipment to the pharmacy. Clean syringes and needles should be supplied at approximately the same rate as used equipment is returned.
4. Contaminated syringes and needles should only be accepted for disposal in a properly designed 'sharps' disposal container. Pharmacists should only take part in a scheme where these containers are available. These should be provided by either the health authority or health board who should also arrange for their collection and disposal at regular intervals.
5. Clients should be encouraged to sheath or otherwise enclose needles before returning them to a pharmacy. The returned equipment should not be handled by anyone other than the person wishing to dispose of it, and that person should be asked to place it in the 'sharps' disposal bin. This disposal bin should be stored well away from customers in a designated area of the pharmacy and in a place known to staff, but where they will not have inadvertent contact with the contaminated waste material.

6. Used contaminated material should ideally be brought to the pharmacy by clients in a personal sealed 'sharps' container. Such containers are now widely available.

7. Staff should be carefully instructed about the risk of needlestick injuries, infection and surface contamination. All enquiries should be referred to the pharmacist. It is important that pharmacists consider having themselves and their staff vaccinated against hepatitis. Such vaccination is free of charge to those health workers involved in contact with drug abusers.

8. Extra caution should be exercised in supplies to children under the age of 16 years. Such clients should normally be referred to a specialist agency.

9. Pharmacists should comply with these guidelines and any additional local protocols issued in respect of the particular scheme in which they are participating.

10. Pharmacists are reminded of the need for confidentiality, and are referred to the Obligations of Principle 4 of the Code of Ethics. Pharmacy staff must be made aware of the importance of confidentiality when dealing with clients requesting clean syringes and needles.

Appendix B

Heroin reefers – a protocol

This document has been prepared for issue as guidance from the Royal Pharmaceutical Society of Great Britain for those pharmacists involved in the preparation and supply of cigarettes impregnated with heroin or other drugs.

Heroin reefers are cigarettes impregnated with a specified dose of diamorphine hydrochloride BP. Reefers are also used on occasions as the vehicle for other drugs of abuse such as methadone hydrochloride, cocaine hydrochloride and amphetamines, the method of preparation being similar for each.

Heroin reefers are prepared by dissolving the prescribed dose of diamorphine hydrochloride BP in a solvent, usually chloroform, and injecting a precisely measured volume of that solution into the tobacco end of each cigarette to give the dose specified by the prescriber. The solvent evaporates leaving the heroin inside the cigarettes. The process discolours the cigarette paper. Once dry the reefers can be dispensed to the patient in a skillet with a dispensing label. The principal benefit to the addict of delivering heroin in the form of a reefer is avoidance of the damage resulting from and associated with intravenous drug administration. As the tobacco burns the heat of combustion sublimes the diamorphine. Any diamorphine vapour which condenses on the cooler tobacco is resublimed as the cigarette burns down. The prescribed daily dose of medication is titrated by the physician according to the patient's habit and is varied by adjusting the number of reefers to be used per day.

The normal practice of prescribers is to instruct the patient to take sufficient cigarettes to the pharmacist in plenty of time to prepare the reefers for dispensing on the authorised day of supply. The Society would not consider it unethical for a pharmacist to supply cigarettes impregnated with heroin in response to a prescription.

Any pharmacy electing to dispense heroin reefers to patients should maintain good contact with the prescribing clinic and be prepared to become involved in counselling of those clients. On a practical point this is necessary to ensure that patients understand the commitments required from them: providing the cigarettes in good time for the preparation of their reefers, knowing when to call in to collect their supplies, storage, safety and other considerations.

The following protocol is issued as guidance to all pharmacists involved in the preparation and supply of reefers impregnated with heroin or other drugs.

PROTOCOL FOR PHARMACISTS WHO PREPARE AND SUPPLY HEROIN REEFERS

Equipment

- Fume cupboard
  The volatile and toxic nature of chloroform makes it necessary for a pharmacist producing reefers to have access to a fume cupboard Id. A DIY type, if properly made, is quite acceptable. (It must be remembered that chloroform is subject to the restrictions of the COSHH regulations.)
- A 1 ml or 2 ml Luer mount glass insulin syringe with an all steel hypodermic needle.

  Note: Do not use plastic disposable syringes or plastic mount needles as these are soluble in chloroform.

- Accurate measuring equipment.
- Facilities for secure storage until collection.

  Note: Heroin reefers are Controlled Drugs and must be stored in a CD cabinet or a safe which has been approved for such a use by the police and a certificate issued.

Personnel

Pharmacists or dispensing assistants directly involved in the manufacture of heroin reefers should receive basic training to ensure accuracy of dispensing and should ideally undergo training about substance misuse/drug abuse plus first-aid training.

Written procedures

A pharmacy providing this service should have a copy of the written procedure for preparation of heroin reefers available for use or inspection by authorised persons.

The basic procedure should be along the following lines:

Background

- 60 mg of heroin by reefer has been determined to be an acceptable therapeutic dose. While the heroin is soluble in water it is much more soluble in chloroform. The latter is the solvent of choice as it evaporates readily at room temperature. Aqueous solutions have been tried but are not recommended as delivery vehicles because of the problems associated with the drying process.

■   A 0.25 ml dose volume of solution per reefer is practicable and is sufficient to stain the cigarette paper characteristically.

Practical

■   Decide the total number of reefers to be made in the dispensing operation.

■   Multiply that number of reefers by the dose prescribed to give the total weight in milligrams of diamorphine hydrochloride required.

■   Multiply the number to be manufactured by 0.25 ml to give the total volume of solution in millilitres.

■   Dissolve all of the diamorphine in sufficient of the chloroform and then make up to volume. Mix well.

■   Each 0.25 ml of the solution will then contain the prescribed dose of diamorphine hydrochloride.

■   Inject the dose volume (0.25 ml) into the tobacco end of each cigarette, placing the bolus approximately 10 mm from the end.

Note: Suitable holders for cigarettes should be used for the injection process to prevent possibility of self injection by the operator.

■   The prepared reefers will need to be left in the fume cupboard until dry. They should be placed into skillets or other suitable container, labelled to comply with the labelling regulations and identify the particular patient for whom the supply is intended. They must not be dispensed when wet.

Any written procedure should also identify the steps to be taken in that pharmacy for ensuring that batches for specific patients are kept separate and that there would be no opportunity or chance of batches being mixed.

Storage/security

A pharmacy involved in the production of heroin reefers will often hold a considerably greater quantity of diamorphine on the premises than most. This, combined with the fact that many addicts may be attending for daily pick-ups, can lead to a security problem both for the premises and for the personnel. Much of the perceived problem can be alleviated by forward planning and adequate documentation of procedures to be followed. The police drug squad officer will usually be able to advise appropriately during his routine visits.

All batches of prepared reefers will need to be labelled and stored in a manner complying with the safe custody regulations under the Misuse of Drugs Act 1971.

The dispensary should be set out to minimise observation by addicts, to prevent access to that part of the premises where the preparation takes place and to safeguard the security of staff.

Record/logging procedure

With the possibility of large quantities of diamorphine being handled, it is essential to balance stocks against supplies regularly. It is suggested that a weekly balance be instituted. A recommended method for smallish quantities is the 'elapsed reefer number' method.

The weight of diamorphine purchased during the week or month is already recorded in the purchases side of the CD Register. This data is matched with the product of the number of reefers dispensed and the strength of each one during the same period. By multiplying those two numbers together the weight dispensed is given. Purchases and supplies are then compared and a trial balance made.

The method is as follows: in the case of a large producer the purchase quantities will be in multiples of 25 g. For smaller producers it will be in multiples of 2 g. Using the former example each 25 g pot of heroin will make a total of 416×60 mg reefers. By marking off the register when a new pot is opened, it is possible to check that approximately 416 reefers have been manufactured from that pot by the time it is empty.

It has been found beneficial to enter the amounts supplied by the number of 60 mg reefers dispensed, e.g. 14×60 mg. By using this method, it is quite simple to add up the number of reefers dispensed until, say, 416 have been dispensed. It is good practice to rule a line across the register either partially or fully to identify this datum point.

Rough calculations at half way points are possible and will identify any significant losses. Where diamorphine is used in other preparations the quantity used should be taken into account when calculating the number of reefers prepared per pot (see Appendix 1).

Prescriptions

Dispensing must be in accordance with correctly written prescriptions. Such prescriptions for heroin reefers must comply with the Misuse of Drugs Regulations and records be kept accordingly in the Controlled Drugs register (see Appendix 2 and 3). When dispensed, reefers should be placed in a suitable container or skillet and a full dispensing label attached for each supply made.

Appearance of reefers

Reefers should be distinguishable from ordinary cigarettes so that there could be no possibility of their being reimpregnated. In practice, the characteristic staining of the cigarette paper suffices. It should not be possible for a patient to mistake a heroin reefer for a normal cigarette and inadvertently allow it to come into the hands of another person.

Inspector

Pharmacists engaging in the preparation of reefers are recommended to contact the Society's inspector, who can offer advice and assistance on the institution of safe working practices.

Liaison with drug dependency clinics

Any pharmacies involved in such supplies should liaise closely with the prescriber and staff at the drug dependency clinics.

Liaison with local drug squad police officers

There should be close liaison with drug squad police officers in the area and pharmacies wishing to become engaged in reefer production should inform the drug squad and the Society's inspector.

'Specials' manufacturers

Some pharmacies may choose to use a specials manufacturer to prepare the reefers. This will obviously involve greater lead times which should be taken into account. It may be necessary to persuade prescribers to issue prescriptions several days in advance of the first day of supply. The prepared reefer is a Controlled Drug and needs to be entered into the register as usual.

Appendix C

Glossary

Acid: LSD

Adam: ecstasy

AKA: ecstasy

Angel dust: phencyclidine

Backtrack: to draw back the plunger of a syringe when injecting, so that blood enters the barrel

Barbs: barbiturates

Base: free cocaine base

Bhang: cannabis

Binge: repeated administration of an intoxicating substance several times in a short space of time. Typically applies to cocaine or alcohol

Blasted: under the influence of drugs

Blow: (1) cannabis (usual definition). (2) to smoke a drug

Blowout: to miss a vein when injecting

Bombed: intoxicated

Bong: home-made smoking apparatus which allows smoke to bubble through water

Bud: cannabis

Bummer: bad trip

Busted: caught using drugs

Buzz: an intense, sudden euphoria which can occur very soon after administering a drug

Charlie: cocaine hydrochloride

Chasing the dragon: the heating of heroin and inhalation of the resultant vapour

China white: alpha-methylfentanyl

Clean: not using, or not in possession of, drugs

Coke: cocaine hydrochloride

Cold turkey: when described as 'doing cold turkey', an individual is undergoing drug withdrawal. The term is most commonly applied to heroin withdrawal

Coming down: the gradual termination of a period of intoxication

Cooking up: preparing injection by heating powdered drug with water

Crack: free cocaine base

Crank: methamphetamine

Crap: poor quality drug

Crash: acute post-intoxication dysphoria

Crystal: methamphetamine. 'Crystals' has also been used to describe amphetamine

Cutting: the diluting of a powdered drug with another powder which may, or may not, be pharmacologically active

Dike: Diconal

DOM: an amphetamine derivative

Dope: usually understood to refer to cannabis in the UK. In the USA more often used to describe heroin

Doves: ecstasy tablets, which may have a bird motif

Downers: sedating drugs, usually barbiturates

Draw: cannabis

Dud or Dummy: poor quality drug containing little or no active ingredient

Ecstasy: 3,4-methylenedioxymethamphetamine, an amphetamine derivative

Eve: 3,4-methylenedioxyethamphetamine or MDEA

Fix: the administration, and subsequent effects, of a psychoactive substance, usually by injection

Flake: cocaine hydrochloride

Flying or In flight: experiencing intoxication

Freebasing: the converting of cocaine hydrochloride to base cocaine, followed by vaporisation then inhalation

Ganja: cannabis

GBH: gamma hydroxybutyrate

Gear: injection equipment

Get off on: experience pleasurable effects from a drug

Grass: cannabis

H: heroin

Hard stuff: heroin

Hash or hashish: cannabis resin

Hash oil: concentrated hashish

Hash plant: cannabis plant

Hemp: cannabis

Herb: cannabis

High: an intense, sudden euphoria which can occur very soon after administering a drug

Hit: (1) a dose of drug. (2) a drug purchase

Hitting up: injecting a drug

Horse: heroin

Hot knifing: the passing of a heated knife through cannabis resin to release vapours which are inhaled

Huffing: inhaling volatile substances from a plastic bag

Ice: methamphetamine

Jammed up: overdosed

Joint: home-made cigarettes containing psychoactive drugs. Most often applied to cigarettes containing heroin or cannabis

Junk: heroin

Junkie: regular heroin user

K: ketamine

Kick: pleasurable feeling from taking a drug

Kit: injection equipment

Kit-kat: ketamine

Liquid X: gamma hydroxybutyrate

Line: powdered cocaine hydrochloride or amphetamine laid out ready to snort

Lung: flexible plastic smoking apparatus which when squeezed enables smoke held within it to be forcibly ejected

Main-lining: the process of injecting

M and M's: ecstasy

Marijuana or marihuana: largely synonymous with cannabis. Usually used at street level to describe the dried flowering heads of the plant

Mary Jane: cannabis

MDA: 3,4-methylenedioxyamphetamine

MDEA: 3,4-methylenedioxyethamphetamine

MDMA: 3,4-methylenedioxymethamphetamine or ecstasy

Meth: methamphetamine

Microdot: dose of LSD in a very small tablet

Moonshine: illicitly distilled concentrated alcoholic drink

Nine ounce block: common size for a large block of hashish

Nuggets: cocaine

OD: overdose

Outfit: injection equipment

PCP: phencyclidine

Poppers: alkyl nitrites

Popping: the injecting of drugs subcutaneously

Pot: cannabis

Puff: cannabis

Pusher: an individual who sells drugs

Rave: a party or event where non-stop music and dancing occur

Reefers: home-made cigarettes containing psychoactive drugs. Most often applied to cigarettes containing heroin or cannabis

Roach: butt of a cannabis cigarette

Rock: free cocaine base

Roid rage: violent outbursts of aggression associated with use of anabolic steroids

Run: repeated administration of an intoxicating substance several times in a short space of time. Typically applies to cocaine

Rush: (1) an intense, sudden euphoria which can occur very soon after administering a drug. (2) a generic name for poppers. (3) a brand name under which butyl nitrite is sold

Score: to buy drugs

Shit: cannabis

Shooting gallery: place where drugs are commonly injected

Shooting-up: the process of injecting

Sinsemilla: variety of hashish containing particularly high concentration of THC. Derived from unfertilised female plants

Skag: heroin

Skagging: the taking of heroin, usually by vaporisation

Skunk: cannabis containing a particularly high concentration of THC, due to selective cultivation

Sleepers: sedative drugs, usually barbiturates

Smack: heroin

Smashed: intoxicated

Smoke: cannabis

Snorting: the inhalation of dry powdered drug into the nose

Snow: cocaine hydrochloride

Spaced out: intoxicated

Special K: ketamine

Speed: amphetamine

Speedball: mixed injection of cocaine hydrochloride and heroin

Spiked: (1) drug adulterated with another psychoactive substance. (2) injected

Spliff: home-made cigarettes containing psychoactive drugs. Most often applied to cigarettes containing heroin or cannabis

Stacking: the use of more than one anabolic steroid at the same time

Stoned: intoxicated (often with cannabis)

Sulph: amphetamine

Super K: ketamine

Synthetic heroin: illicit fentanyl derivatives

Tab: tablet

Tems: temazepam

TMF: 3-methylfentanyl, a synthetic opioid

Tranx: benzodiazepines, especially temazepam

Trip: an intoxicating experience

Trips: LSD

Uppers: any stimulant drug, but usually amphetamine

Vitamin K: ketamine

Wash: free cocaine base

Wasted: under the influence of drugs

Weed: cannabis

Whiz: amphetamine

Works: injection equipment: *i.e.* needle and syringe

Wrap: folded card or paper containing powdered drug such as heroin or amphetamine

Wrecked: intoxicated

XTC: ecstasy

Appendix D

Sources of further information and advice

ALCOHOL

Accept: Ethnic Alcohol Counselling
Holdsworth House, Staines Road, Middlesex TW3 3HU
Tel (0181) 577 6059

Accept Services UK
724 Fulham Road, London SW6 5SE
Tel (0171) 371 7477
Group therapy organisation encouraging abstinence

Al-Anon Family Groups
61 Great Dover Street, London SE1 4YF
Tel (0171) 403 0888
Supports families affected by alcoholism; 24-hour helpline

Alateen
61 Great Dover Street, London SE1 4YF
Tel (0171) 403 0888
Supports teenagers who have an alcoholic parent; 24-hour helpline

Alcoholics Anonymous
PO Box 514, 11 Redcliffe Gardens, London SW10 9BQ
Tel (0171) 352 9779
PO Box 1, Stonebow House, Stonebow, York YO1 2NJ
Tel (01904) 644026

Alcohol Concern
305 Gray's Inn Road, London WC1X 8QF
Tel (0171) 833 3471

Alcohol Concern Wales
Brunel House, 2 Fitzalan Road, Cardiff CF2 1ER
Tel (01222) 488000

Drinkwatchers
200 Seagrove Road, London SW16 1RQ
Tel (0171) 381 3155

Medical Council on Alcoholism
1 St Andrew's Place, London NW1 4LB
Tel (0171) 487 4445

Northern Ireland Council on Alcohol
40 Elmwood Avenue, Belfast BT9 6AZ
Tel (01232) 664434

Scottish Council on Alcohol
137–145 Sauchiehall Street, Glasgow G2 3EW
Tel (0141) 333 9677

ANABOLIC STEROIDS

Sports Council
Doping and Control Unit, Walkden House, 3–10 Melton Street, London
NW1 2EB
Tel (0171) 383 5667

BENZODIAZEPINE DEPENDENTS

MIND (National Association for Mental Health)
Granta House, 15–19 Broadway, London E15 4BQ
Tel (0181) 519 2122 or (0181) 522 1728
The major mental health charity in the UK. Also provides support in the field of drug dependence generally

Council for Involuntary Tranquilliser Addiction (CITA)
Cavendish House, Brighton Road, Waterloo, Liverpool L22 5NG
Tel (0151) 949 0102

DRUG ABUSE

Addiction Community Centres
724 Fulham Road, London SW6 5SE
Tel (0171) 371 7477
Provides day treatment centres for drug users and families. Group and individual counselling

ADFAM National
5th Floor, Epworth House, 25 City Road, London EC1Y 1AA
Tel (0171) 638 3700
Provides support to families affected by drug abuse

Department of Health
Produces a range of leaflets including *Drugs: a Parent's Guide* and *Solvents: a Parent's Guide*, as well as a range of other booklets aimed at parents and children or teenagers. These are available free from: Health Publications Unit, Heywood Stores, No.2 Site, Manchester Road, Heywood, Lancashire OL10 2PZ

Drugaid: All Wales Drugline
1 Neville Street, Cardiff CF1 8LP
Tel (01222) 383313
24-hour helpline

Drugline Scotland
Tel (0800) 776 600. Freephone

Drugs Training Project
University of Stirling
Tel (01786) 73171 ext 2774
Offers training and information to participants in drug-related projects in Scotland

Families Anonymous
The Doddington & Rollo Community Association, Charlotte Despard Avenue, Battersea, London SW11 5JE
Tel (0171) 498 4680
Assists families and friends of those with a problem related to drug abuse

Freephone Drug Problems
Dial 100 and ask for Freephone Drug Problems. A recorded message gives the telephone numbers of local drug services throughout the UK

Institute for the Study of Drug Dependence (ISDD)
Waterbridge House, 32–36 Loman Street, London SE1 0EE
Tel (0171) 928 1211
Can provide information to the healthcare professional and lay person alike. A catalogue of publications is available upon request. Also houses a library which can be visited; it can also provide photocopies for which a fee is charged

Narcotics Anonymous
PO Box 1980, London N19 3LS
Tel (0171) 272 9040 or (0171) 730 0009

National Addiction Centre
Addiction Sciences Building, 4 Windsor Walk, London SE5 8AF
Tel (0171) 703 5411

National Drugs Helpline
Tel (0800) 776600
Free and confidential 24-hour service. Can provide information about drug abuse to users, those worried about friends or relatives that use drugs

Northern Ireland Regional Unit
Shaftesbury Square Hospital, 116–122 Great Victoria Street, Belfast BT2 7BG
Tel (01232) 329808
Offers counselling and educational materials, and can provide details of local services in Northern Ireland

Release
388 Old Street, London EC1N 9LT
Tel (0171) 729 9904 [Mon-Fri 10am to 6pm]
Tel (0171) 603 8654 [24-hour emergency number]
Offers advice on drugs and legal matters

Scottish Drugs Forum
5 Oswald Street, Glasgow G1 5QR
Tel (0141) 221 1175
Co-ordinates services to drug abusers in Scotland

Standing Conference on Drug Abuse (SCODA)
Waterbridge House, 32–36 Loman Street, London SE1 0EE
Tel (0171) 928 9500
The national body which advises the government. Membership is open to those who work with drug abusers. Provides information on local services and training

TACADE (The Advisory Council on Alcohol and Drug Education)
1 Hulme Place, The Crescent, Salford M5 4QA
Tel (0161) 745 8925
Provides educational and training material

Turning Point
New Loom House, 101 Backchurch Lane, London E1 1LU
Tel (0171) 702 2300
Provides rehabilitation, counselling and care for drugs abusers and their families

TOBACCO SMOKING

Action on Smoking and Health (ASH)
109 Gloucester Place, London W1H 3PH
Tel (0171) 935 3519

QUIT
102 Gloucester Place, London W1H 3DA
Tel (0171) 487 2858

QUITLINE
Tel (0171) 487 3000

SOLVENT ABUSE

Re-Solv
30a High Street, Stone, Staffordshire ST15 8AW
Tel (01785) 817885
The society for the prevention of solvent and volatile substance abuse. A national charity providing advice and a range of educational materials on volatile substance abuse

OTC MEDICINES

Over-Count
20 Brewery Street, Dumfries, DG1 2RP
Tel (01387) 770404
Advisory service, support and friendship for those dependent on OTC medicines

Index

Page numbers in **bold** indicate a main section on a particular subject in the text or an appendix.